T0325168

Cognitive Enhancement in Schizophrenia and Related Disorders

Cognitive Enhancement in Schizophrenia and Related Disorders

Matcheri Keshavan
Harvard Medical School

Shaun Eack
University of Pittsburgh

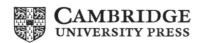
CAMBRIDGE
UNIVERSITY PRESS

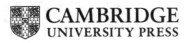

Shaftesbury Road, Cambridge CB2 8EA, United Kingdom

One Liberty Plaza, 20th Floor, New York, NY 10006, USA

477 Williamstown Road, Port Melbourne, VIC 3207, Australia

314–321, 3rd Floor, Plot 3, Splendor Forum, Jasola District Centre, New Delhi – 110025, India

103 Penang Road, #05–06/07, Visioncrest Commercial, Singapore 238467

Cambridge University Press is part of Cambridge University Press & Assessment, a department of the University of Cambridge.

We share the University's mission to contribute to society through the pursuit of education, learning and research at the highest international levels of excellence.

www.cambridge.org
Information on this title: www.cambridge.org/9781107194786

DOI: 10.1017/9781108163682

First published 2019

A catalogue record for this publication is available from the British Library

ISBN   978-1-107-19478-6   Hardback

This book is dedicated to
Gerard E. Hogarty, M.S.W. (1935–2006)

Contents

Foreword

Professor Dame Til Wykes, Institute of Psychiatry, Psychology and Neuroscience, King's College London SE5 8AF

People diagnosed with schizophrenia have multiple problems including their obvious delusions and hallucinations, their positive symptoms. Even after the acute problems have subsided, there are still other difficulties that impair functioning, particularly in social relationships, employment, and in achieving their personal goals. Although we have treatments for the obvious symptoms, we now know that the cognitive problems are key drivers of these functional and personal achievements. However, it has taken many years to be optimistic about their alleviation. It was thought that the difficulties were traits that made individuals vulnerable to disorder and were immutable, but we now know that we can help to remediate these thinking skills by providing cognitive rehabilitation. This book covers the history, the emergence of optimism and the theory that drove therapy developments. Although I may disagree with some of the levels of theory description, I do not disagree with the description of how cognitive enhancement therapy was built and its importance amid the panoply of therapy options. Its ambitions are wide and the ingredients varied.

The scientific literature is littered with, in my view, spurious arguments about whether cognitive training needs to be top-down, bottom-up, or compensatory, but this is not even attended to by cognitive enhancement because it covers all the bases. It includes specific cognitive training with practice (bottom-up) for the development of strategies for efficient problem solving (top-down) and then combines all these with an adaptation of the environment (compensatory) to reduce the need for speed of processing or flexibility in approaches to problems. This method also includes therapeutic inputs to guide the process of therapy and assessment so the individuals are not overwhelmed. This is what makes it a therapy rather than "brain training," because the therapist allows more personalized therapy, can increase motivation, and importantly help link therapy goals to personal real-world goals.

The development of the best cognitive treatments has undoubtedly been hindered by the personal prejudices of its proponents. This book lays out all the available options which allow a clinician to take their choice but also points out the similarities despite their different names and marketing. The book also points to the embedding of this sort of therapy among other tools including medication.

The most powerful part of the book is the transfer of expert clinical experience from the authors to readers. This information is clearly set out to empower those who are embarking on providing therapy. There is an emphasis on personalisation along with the development of a good therapeutic alliance. Both are vital to engaging individuals and are often a therapeutic hurdle, especially for a group that has often experienced multiple failures.

When I was asked to write this foreword I thought I would be able to produce a reasonable draft in a few days but little did I know how interesting the book would be. Delving into it was just not enough, I read it from cover to cover. This is clearly the book I was meaning to write and I am very pleased that Drs. Keshavan and Eack have now written it as it certainly takes the pressure off me.

In conclusion, cognitive enhancement in its many forms can improve thinking skills and has benefits for functioning. This book is a stepping stone to encourage its use more widely. But we should not assume that the provision of this therapy is the sole determiner of achieving personal goals. Society still discriminates against individuals who have mental illnesses, and the associated stigma affects the individuals and their families. We all hope that better recovery outcomes will follow the introduction of cognitive enhancement and contribute to therapeutic optimism that will stimulate the beneficial changes in society and open up further opportunities for our patients.

Preface

Schizophrenia and related psychotic disorders are among the most disabling illnesses in all of medicine. While acute psychotic symptoms are manageable by current medication treatments, the persistent deficits in cognition which underlie functional disability remain poorly addressed. Psychotherapeutic treatments remain the mainstay of our efforts in addressing these roadblocks to recovery. The authors of this volume came together with their abiding interests in contributing to this serious treatment gap and in no small measure due to the important influence and mentorship of Gerard E. Hogarty (1935–2006), who pioneered the field of cognitive enhancement in schizophrenia and who continues to inspire our own thinking on the topic. In our decade-long collaborations both as clinicians and researchers we have come to appreciate the substantial advances as well as challenges in understanding cognition, brain plasticity, and therapeutic interventions in neuropsychiatry, notably in schizophrenia. We are also optimistic for the advances that the future holds in this field and felt that a summary of the current state of cognitive enhancement in schizophrenia and related disorders would be a valuable contribution to practitioners, educators, and researchers.

While cognitive impairments characterize many psychiatric disorders, this book focuses on schizophrenia because this is the field of our own expertise. We believe, however, that the principles in this book would be applicable to other related major psychiatric disorders as well. Schizophrenia is a spectrum of disorders (such as schizoaffective disorder and psychotic affective disorders) in which cognitive difficulties are core features, persistent, and life-long. Further, even though cognitive health is a primary focus of this volume, we appreciate the importance of alterations in emotion and behavior that are integral to these conditions and necessitate an integrated approach with other psychosocial and pharmacological interventions. We prefer the term cognitive enhancement to terms such as cognitive remediation or cognitive rehabilitation, because of the former's broader scope and its non-stigmatizing nature.

This book is designed to serve the needs of practicing clinicians, students of mental health and researchers. Patients and family members may find this book helpful as well. We have adopted a somewhat conversational style wherever possible, interspersing our personal experiences and value systems in caring for patients with schizophrenia with what we are learning from decades of systematic research. We have focused more on Cognitive Enhancement Therapy (CET), originally developed by Hogarty and colleagues, in which we have the most experience. We have also described several other approaches to cognitive interventions. We have used ample illustrations, mostly originally developed, case illustrations largely from our practice, and an up-to-date bibliography of the major works in this field. The text begins with a basic principles section, with overviews of our current understanding of cognition and its impairment in schizophrenia, of the nature of brain plasticity in health and disease, and of the history and principles underlying cognitive enhancement. The second section is on the approaches to cognitive enhancement. It begins with an overview of engagement and stabilization early in the course of schizophrenia, which is a key prerequisite to successful cognitive enhancement approaches. We then provide a detailed summary of strategies to enhance neurocognition and social cognition using computer-based, individual, and group interventions. We end this section with an overview of pharmacotherapy for schizophrenia including an account of the limited data on the pharmacological enhancement of cognition. In the final section, we focus on how to optimize and personalize cognitive interventions to the individual patient. The last chapter concludes with our perspectives on the current state of the field and where it should be headed, in terms of research and implementation of cognitive enhancement in routine clinical settings.

It is important to note that this book is not designed or intended to serve as a treatment manual for Cognitive Enhancement Therapy or other cognitive interventions, but potential users will find this text a significant resource in their work to learn about and implement these interventions into their practice. The definitive treatment manual for Cognitive Enhancement Therapy (Hogarty & Greenwald, 2006) is available separately from those authors at www.CognitiveEnhancementTherapy.com and should be relied upon as the primary resource for learning that approach. We have taken care to refer readers to the primary texts of other interventions discussed throughout this book as well. If the practice principles in this book do not appear to apply to or are counter the situation presented by any individual patient or clinical situation, the practitioner should use his/her clinical judgment, and/or seek an appropriate referral. We will be gratified if this book serves to provide guidance, confidence, and understanding to care providers who work with persons living with schizophrenia and their family members.

Acknowledgments

We are grateful to several individuals who made this contribution possible. Drs. Michelle Friedman-Yakoobian, Synthia Guimond, Asha Keshavan, Emily Kline, Raquelle Mesholam Gately, Luis Sandoval, and William Stone provided valuable comments. Jayne-Marie Nova was instrumental in meticulously creating the bibliography. We also appreciate the support, patience, and understanding by our spouses, Asha Keshavan and Ashley B. Eack. Vinod Srihari meticulously reviewed the manuscript, and provided valuable edits and suggestions.

Cognition and Its Impairment in Schizophrenia and Related Psychotic Disorders

1.1 Introduction

This chapter provides an overview of the diverse aspects of human cognition, including non-social cognitive functions such as attention, executive function, and memory and social cognitive functions such as emotion recognition and perspective taking. We review the nature of these functions, how they are impaired in schizophrenia and related disorders, and how to assess them. We then outline an evolving understanding of the brain circuitries underlying these functions. A detailed review of this vast literature is beyond the scope of this chapter, but we here summarize the key points a practitioner of cognitive enhancement approaches needs to keep in mind.

Emil Kraepelin (Figure 1.1), considered the father of modern psychiatry, pointed out that cognitive impairments are among the core manifestations of dementia praecox, a term originally introduced by Morel. Dementia praecox was later termed schizophrenia by Eugen Bleuler, a Swiss psychiatrist who viewed this as a group of illnesses with diverse causes which had its central feature as a "splitting" of mental functions (schism in Latin means splitting). Kraepelin described a wide range of cognitive difficulties in dementia praecox including impairments in attention, learning, and problem solving and noted the impact of these changes for independent living, social, and occupational functioning (Kraepelin, Barclay, & Robertson, 1919). However, the centrality of cognitive impairments in schizophrenia was largely ignored till the middle of the last century, perhaps because of the dominance of psychodynamic conceptualizations of this illness. Modern neuropsychological conceptualizations of psychotic disorders began in the 1950s and 1960s (Broadbent, 1958; Hemsley, 1977; McGhie & Chapman, 1961). Cognition has been continuously and extensively studied in schizophrenia over the past several decades using a wide range of traditional Neuropsychological tasks as well as paradigms developed from cognitive neuroscience and experimental psychology.

Case Study 1.1

Jeffrey is a 26-year-old single unemployed man living with his parents. He had been diagnosed with schizoaffective disorder six years ago when he first began, during his second year of college, to experience paranoid and grandiose delusions as well as auditory hallucinations. He had begun believing that he is destined to become the President of the United States and that he was being monitored by the FBI and the CIA so that he would be "vetted" and groomed to the highest office.

Jeffrey had an unremarkable childhood, except that his early milestones were slightly delayed. He started speaking at the age of 2. He did well academically in middle school but had been evaluated by a psychologist for a possible attention deficit disorder. His grades began to decline during high school and his grades were mostly Cs by his junior year. He began college after high school but had to take a break during his first year because of academic difficulties, as well as increasing anxiety and feelings that he had more important missions in life than just getting a college degree. He could not concentrate, and could not organize his class schedules. He started becoming socially withdrawn, spending a great deal of time on Twitter where he began to post garbled political messages. It is at this time that he was hospitalized for his first psychotic episode.

Over the past 4 years, Jeffrey has been hospitalized on three occasions and he is now an outpatient at a university psychiatry clinic. His symptoms have improved but he intermittently relapses because of his poor compliance with medications (risperidone, valproate, and benztropine) as well as his forgetfulness. He does not believe that he has any illness and he is not concerned that others do not share his beliefs about his delusions; he has been unable to date or have significant friendships because his "presidential" delusions come up prominently early in his conversation. While he has been able to get job interviews, he has not been able to hold a job for longer than a few months. Jeffrey has a slow processing speed, as evidenced by performance at the 25th percentile on the BACS Symbol Coding test of the MATRICs battery (described later in this chapter). His attention is poor, as reflected by scores at the 10th percentile on the Trail Making Test - Part A and the CPT-IP. His working memory (WMS-3 Spatial Span test) was also in the low average (25th) percentile. He performed in the average range (40th percentile) on spatial reasoning (NAB Mazes test). He scored in the 20th percentile on the Managing Emotions subtest of the MSCEIT (social cognition).

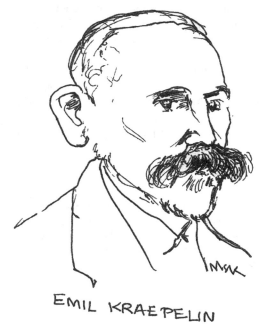

Figure 1.1 Emil Kraepelin (1856–1926), considered by many to be the father of modern psychiatry, first described dementia praecox, later termed schizophrenia

EMIL KRAEPELIN

As this chapter will reveal, cognitive impairments are a core aspect of schizophrenia. An important point to remember is that schizophrenia involves impairment not just in any one of these cognitive domains, but usually a combination of many deficits; the degree to which any one domain is impaired might differ between patients, and may also differ by illness phase (Heinrichs & Zakzanis, 1998; Mesholam-Gately et al., 2009). The above patient narrative (see box) illustrates this point, and highlights how these impairments substantively affect day-to-day functioning.

1.2 Nature of Cognitive Deficits in Schizophrenia

Cognitive Impairments are Highly Prevalent in Schizophrenia

Although cognitive deficits are a core aspect of schizophrenia, many patients may appear to have normal cognitive function. In healthy individuals, cognitive function is strongly predicted by parental levels of education. Studies suggest that the majority of patients (>90%) perform at below what would be expected from the parental level of education (Keefe, Eesley, & Poe, 2005), while positive and negative symptoms are present in about half to two-thirds of patients at any point in time (Figure 1.2). Thus, almost all schizophrenia patients have some degree of cognitive impairment relative to what their level of cognitive function would have been if they had never developed the illness. Over 90% of patients have impairments in at least one domain and about 75% have deficits in two domains. Cognitive impairments in schizophrenia also are more severe than in affective disorders (Hill et al., 2013).

Cognitive Impairments May Precede the Illness, and Might Represent Premorbid Hallmarks of Schizophrenia

First degree relatives of patients with schizophrenia have cognitive impairments, albeit at a milder level, about a half a standard deviation below healthy populations (Keshavan

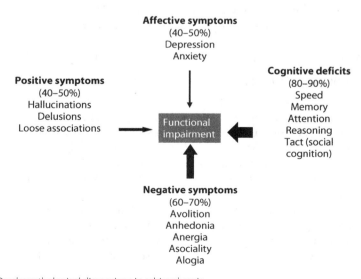

Figure 1.2 Psychopathological dimensions in schizophrenia

et al., 2010; Liu et al., 2015a). Over 90% of monozygotic twins discordant for schizophrenia have cognitive impairments (Goldberg et al., 1990). Modest global cognitive deficits are often apparent in early life (premorbid) phases (Woodberry, Giuliano, & Seidman, 2008). Cognitive deficits or decline are also present in individuals at high clinical risk for schizophrenia though to a lesser extent than impairments observed in established schizophrenia (Giuliano et al., 2012) and can predict the conversion to psychosis (Seidman et al., 2010).

Cognitive Impairments Predict Functional Outcome

Cognitive functioning reliably predicts functional outcome in schizophrenia. Functional outcome refers to independent living, as well as occupational and social functioning. Effect sizes of the relationship between cognition and outcome are medium for specific domains and larger for composite scores (Green, 2000). A meta-analysis has shown that social cognition may explain more variance in functional outcome than nonsocial cognition (Fett et al., 2011). Social cognition may be a mediator of the relationship between neurocognition and functional outcome (Couture, Penn, & Roberts, 2006). Overall, impaired cognition is a rate limiting factor for successful functional recovery.

Cognitive Impairments Persist during the Course of the Illness, and are a Trait Aspect of the Illness

Cognitive impairments are reliably and broadly seen by the first psychotic episode, tend to persist at the same or slightly increased level of deficit, and are most prominent in verbal declarative memory and processing speed (Mesholam-Gately et al., 2009). Cognitive impairments show some inconsistent relationships with negative symptoms and positive symptoms of the disorder (Bozikas et al., 2004). While psychotic symptoms fluctuate over the course of time cognitive difficulties rarely do (Figure 1.3). In general, the nature and severity of cognitive impairments are not explained by antipsychotic medications with the exception of anticholinergics (Wojtalik et al., 2012). The level of neurocognitive impairments tends to remain stable during adult life (Rund, 1998).

Cognitive Impairments in Schizophrenia are Pervasive and Span Several Domains

Several meta-analyses have suggested that a wide range of cognitive functions are impaired in schizophrenia, at a moderate to severe degree, with effect sizes varying from the medium-to-large range (Heinrichs & Zakzanis, 1998; Mesholam-Gately et al., 2009). Notably, impaired cognitive domains include psychomotor Speed, working Memory, verbal memory and learning, Attention, Reasoning and executive functions, and Tactfulness or Social cognition; the acronym SMARTS can be used to summarize the key domains for teaching purposes.

We outline below the most important cognitive domains that are impaired in schizophrenia. Some cognitive functions, such as procedural memory, implicit learning and visual perceptual skills may be less involved (Gold et al., 2009). It is possible that the islands of preserved cognitive capability in schizophrenia may be capitalized for

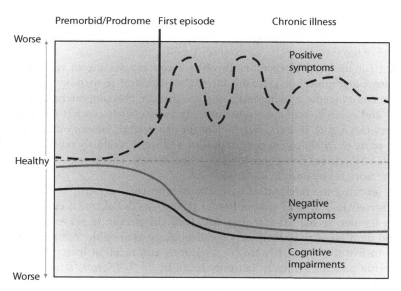

Figure 1.3 Course of cognitive impairment (black, lower line), negative (grey, lower line) and positive symptoms (black, top line) in schizophrenia.

cognitive remediation using the principles of compensatory neuroplasticity, as discussed in Chapter 2 of this volume.

1.3 Non-Social Cognition Deficits in Schizophrenia

Speed of Processing

Patients with schizophrenia have significant impairments in speed of information processing (Morrens, Hulstijn, & Sabbe, 2006). A common test that taps into this domain is the Digit Symbol Coding task, which is part of the various editions of the Wechsler intelligence scales. The task requires the participant to substitute a series of numbers to symbol as rapidly as possible (e.g. within 90 seconds). Deficits in processing speed are significantly correlated with activities of daily life, occupational functioning as well as social functioning. Psychomotor speed may also be impaired by sedative antipsychotic medications, benzodiazepines and mood stabilizers.

Memory

Broadly, memory is considered to include multiple processes. First is the working memory, which refers to the ability to hold a limited amount of information "on-line" for a short period of time, like a mental "scratch-pad." A typical test for this cognitive domain is the Digit Span forward task (repeating a string of digits) and backward task (which requires the information to be held online as well as reordered) in the Wechsler intelligence scales. Schizophrenia patients show impairments in these tasks (Goldman-Rakic, 1994). Another common type of test is the n-back task, in which a sequence of stimuli are presented and the subject has to indicate when the new stimulus (e.g. a number or letter) matches the one from n stimuli earlier in the sequence; n can be adjusted to vary the difficulty level of the task.

Explicit (or declarative) memory involves a conscious sense of remembering and recall of autobiographical or factual information. Declarative memory is of two types: semantic memory (remembering facts, such as what are the components of a thanksgiving meal) and episodic memory (remembering events, such as what one had for dinner the previous night). By contrast, implicit (or procedural) memory does not involve a conscious sense of recall; an example of the latter is not consciously recalling the steps of how to ride a bicycle but being able to do so when needed. There is no clear evidence that implicit memory is impaired in schizophrenia.

Verbal learning and retrieval, as well as recognition of previously learnt material, are all substantively impaired in schizophrenia (Heinrichs & Zakzanis, 1998). Commonly used tests involve verbal list learning, in which the person is presented with 12–16 words, and then asked to immediately recall as many as possible. After repeated learning of up to five times on 16-word lists, controls can recall at least 13 of the words, schizophrenia patients typically can only recall up to 9. There is strong evidence for an association between verbal memory and poor social and vocational outcome in schizophrenia.

Attention

Attention is robustly impaired in schizophrenia. Two aspects of attention are: *sustained attention*, or vigilance which is the ability to maintain a continuous focus on stimuli (such as watching the train arrival times on the monitor to watch for the boarding signal for your destination), and *selective attention* which is the ability to focus on relevant stimuli and ignore competing stimuli. This is what you need in a noisy cocktail party where you have to pay attention to what your friend is saying, while ignoring all the other chatter around you. Continuous Performance Tasks (CPT) are typical tests of *sustained attention* in which a series of stimuli are presented, and the individual has to respond each time to a target stimulus appears (e.g. whenever an X appears after an A). There is evidence of impairments in sustained attention in schizophrenia and bipolar disorder (Heinrichs & Zakzanis, 1998).

Selective attention involves casting a spotlight on relevant external stimuli, or on internal mental representations, and ignoring competing stimuli. This may involve filtering (including desired input but excluding inputs that are not relevant), and categorizing information based on stimulus attributes such as shape or color. A classic test of selective attention is the Stroop task. In this task, the subject is asked to name the colors of the words and not read the words, as fast as he can. Thus, if the word "BLUE" is printed in red, the subject should say "RED." Naming the color of the word takes longer and causes more errors when the color of the ink does not match the name of the color. This Stroop effect is abnormal in schizophrenia (Carter, Robertson, & Nordahl, 1992).

Another aspect of attention, impaired in schizophrenia and other related neuropsychiatric disorders, is *attention capacity*, i.e. the ability to process more than one concurrent task (like having a conversation while driving, and sipping coffee at the same time). Many patients find it difficult to multi-task because of a reduction in attention capacity (Thoma & Daum, 2008).

Reasoning and Problem-Solving

Executive functioning refers to activities such as problem-solving, planning, and shifting between two or more tasks. These abilities are critically important in day-to-day life. A common test that is used is the Wisconsin Card Sorting Test (WCST; see Figure 1.4). In this task (Heaton, 1980), the participant is asked to sort a deck of cards into groups (based on the principle of either color, number, or shape) and has to figure out the rules based on the feedback of the answers being correct or incorrect. The principle will change during the test, and the participant has to figure out the new rules and change his responses accordingly. Performance on this task – which requires conceptual flexibility and an ability to shift mental set – is consistently impaired in schizophrenia (Berman, 1987).

Another aspect of executive function – related to selective attention discussed above – is monitoring of conflict and choosing appropriate responses; a commonly used test for this is the Flanker task. In this task, a series of arrows are presented pointing to the right or left. Participants respond in the direction of the arrow pressing the right button if the arrow points to right in congruent trials while they have to press the left button when presented with a right pointing arrow in incongruent trials.

In general, aspects of "fluid" intelligence (i.e. abilities to process new information, such as working memory and executive function) are more likely to be impaired than "crystalline" intelligence (ability to use already acquired information such as vocabulary) in neuropsychiatric disorders. Both aspects of intelligence are altered in schizophrenia. However, impaired crystallized intelligence can give us a measure of premorbid abilities, while decline in fluid intelligence is likely to reflect disease-related intellectual decline.

1.4 Social Cognition Deficits in Schizophrenia

Social cognition is a composite term used to refer to psychological processes involved in perception, inferring about and responding in social situations (Green et al., 2008). Social cognition involves several components: emotion perception, the ability to take other people's perspectives, and the ability to appraise the social context. Individuals with schizophrenia consistently perform poorly when asked to identify emotional expressions on peoples' faces (Mueser et al., 1997). Schizophrenia patients also show deficits in

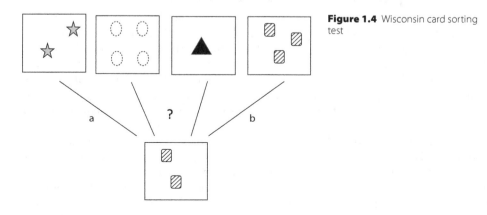

Figure 1.4 Wisconsin card sorting test

perception of emotions in speech and videotaped monologues. Deficits tend to be more prominent in the perception of negative or neutral stimuli than in the perception of positive emotions (one of the authors [MSK] has observed in his practice that on days when he walks into his office with a flat facial expression, patients often ask whether he is angry with them for something!). Indeed, one of our studies has shown that emotion perception to neutral faces is impaired in adolescents at high familial risk for schizophrenia (Eack et al., 2010).

Schizophrenia patients also have difficulty in taking viewpoints of other people *(mentalizing or perspective taking)* and making inferences about their mental states based on available social context information. This process, also called "Theory of Mind" (ToM), underlies the ability to understand hints, intentions, humor, irony, and metaphor. There is some evidence that schizophrenia patients have deficits in humor perception, and this may be related to ToM impairments (Marjoram et al., 2005).

Context appraisal refers to a person's ability to judge social cues from information in the social context, and awareness of the roles, rules, and norms that characterize different, sometimes ambiguous social situations. This includes the ability to perceive social cues (social perception), processing such information and choosing an appropriate response in a given social situation.

Attributional style refers to the way in which one makes sense of social events in life. For example, if a friend does not smile at you during a social encounter, you might assume either that you are deliberately being ignored, or that the friend may not have noticed you. The chosen explanation will clearly decide which way you react emotionally and behaviorally to this situation.

Figure 1.5 illustrates the different components of social cognition. Our patient, Jeffrey, has not been able to hold a job consistently because of his difficulty with several aspects of social cognition. As an example, if one has to navigate a work-related interaction successfully (such as asking for a day off), he has to first assess his boss's mood (emotion recognition), figure out what his boss might be thinking (perspective taking or theory of mind), assess when might be the best time and place to make the request (social context appraisal), and make the appropriate interpretation of boss's response (e.g. a denied request does not automatically mean the boss does not like him). In Chapter 6, we will discuss how cognition enhancement approaches target these aspects of social cognition.

1.5 Metacognition Deficits in Schizophrenia

Metacognition has been defined as "thinking about thinking." This term has been used in several contexts and refers to three broad sets of function: (a) monitoring or evaluation of one's own cognitive functions; (b) regulation of one's own cognition, which includes executive functions and cognitive control; and (c) metacognitive knowledge, i.e. knowledge of the task difficulties, resources needed to tackle them, and alternative approaches to improve cognitive performance (Flavell, 1979). There is evidence for impairments in all of the above aspects of metacognition in schizophrenia; such impairments appear to predict functional outcome (Koren et al., 2006; Lysaker et al., 2014).

A consequence of impaired metacognition is the inability to think about one's own delusional beliefs and the ability to change them in the context of new evidence. It has been suggested that delusions develop as a consequence of cognitive bias and in particular a tendency to "jump to conclusions" (Garety et al., 2013). This reasoning bias has been widely replicated in schizophrenia not only in people with delusions but also in people

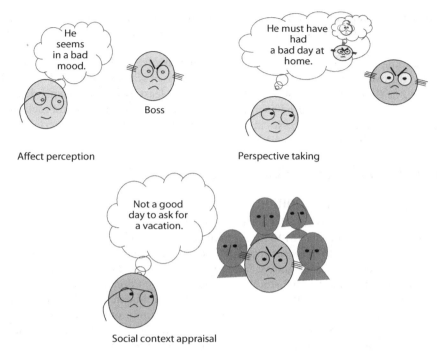

Figure 1.5 Components of social cognition

who have recovered from delusions and individuals at high-risk for psychoses. While the precise mechanisms underlying the *jumping to conclusions* bias remain to be understood, studies suggest that other aspects of cognitive impairment and in particular executive dysfunction may be related to such reasoning biases.

Insight and Illness Appraisal

One of the most common problems in schizophrenia is lack of insight. Insight is a multidimensional concept and includes accurate self-awareness, correct attribution, and recognition of one's own illness and need for treatment. Patients with schizophrenia may have impairment in one or more of these dimensions. It has been found that impaired cognition is strongly related to poor insight in schizophrenia (Keshavan et al., 2004). It has even been suggested that lack of insight in schizophrenia might reflect an anosognosia, a known neurological condition with impaired awareness of one's own neurological disability (Lehrer & Lorenz, 2014).

Foresight

A cognitive function related to insight is foresight, the ability to think of the long-term consequences of one's behavior and use this information to guide present and future actions. Foresight is critically related to functional disability in schizophrenia, as a diminished capacity for recognizing the long-term consequences of one's behavior (which has been called future "myopia"), and would likely have a negative impact on interpersonal relationships in many different domains (e.g. home and work). Indeed, foresight significantly predicted functional outcome in one of our longitudinal studies (Eack & Keshavan, 2008).

In summary, cognitive deficits in schizophrenia involve multiple domains, and are central to the overall psychopathological manifestations of schizophrenia and related disorders. While the core aspects of these illnesses may at least in part be independent, it is likely that they overlap; impaired cognition, deficits in social cognition and metacognition, and affect regulation processes may interact to cause alterations in experiences and beliefs that underlie the pathogenesis of psychosis (Figure 1.6).

1.6 How Do We Assess Cognitive Function?

Assessing Non-Social Cognition

A battery of cognitive tests called the Measurement and Treatment Research to Improve Cognition in Schizophrenia (MATRICS) battery has been developed by the National Institute of Mental Health in recent years for assessment of cognition (Green et al., 2004). The MATRICS Consensus Cognitive Battery (MCCB) is the field-standard for cognitive assessments for clinical trial studies and assesses seven domains of cognitive functions using ten tests (Table 1.1). This battery is easy to administer, has high fidelity, and takes a little over 1 hour to complete on average. In community settings with limited resources however, it may be more practical to use smaller batteries with similar reliability and validity, such as the Brief Assessment of Cognition in Schizophrenia (BACS; Keefe, 2004). The BACS takes about 35 minutes. Both the MCCB and BACS have alternate forms available so that they can be used to minimize practice effects. Other available paper and pencil and computerized test batteries include the Repeatable Battery for the Assessment of Neuropsychological Status (RBANS; Randolph et al., 1998), Cambridge Neuropsychological Test Automated Battery (CANTAB; Sahakian et al., 1988), and the

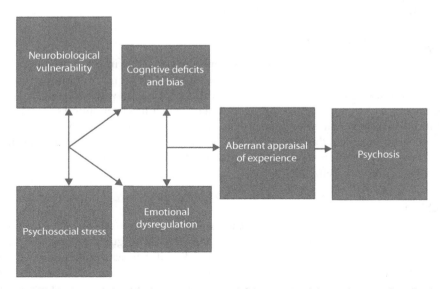

Figure 1.6 The intricate relationships between cognitive deficits, emotional dysregulation, and psychosis

Table 1.1 Neurocognitive tests used in research and clinical settings

Tests	Processing speed	Working memory	Verbal learning/ memory	Visuospatial learning/ memory	Attention	Reasoning/ problem solving	Language	Verbal fluency	Abstract thinking	Social cognition	Admin time (min)	References
Cognitive batteries												
MATRICS	×	×	×	×	×	×				×	60	Neuchterlein et al., 2008
BACS	×	×	×	×		×		×			35	Keefe, 2004
CANTAB	×	×	×	×	×	×				×	60	Barnett et al., 2010
COGSTATE	×	×	×	×	×	×				×	35	Pietrzak et al., 2009
RBANS	×	×	×	×	×		×				25–45	Wilk et al., 2002
MoCA	×	×	×	×	×		×	×	×		10	Wu et al., 2014
Penn CNB	×	×	×	×	×	×	×	×		×	60	Gur et al., 2001
Interview-based												
SCoRS	×	×	×	×	×	×					35	Keefe et al., 2006
CGI-CogS	×	×	×	×	×	×				×	30	Ventura et al., 2008
BRIEF		×				×					10–15	Gioia et al., 2000
CAI	×	×	×		×	×				×	20	Ventura et al., 2010

Abbreviations: MATRICS: Measurement and Treatment Research to Improve Cognition in Schizophrenia; BACS: Brief Assessment of Cognition in Schizophrenia; CANTAB: Cambridge Neuropsychological Test Automated Battery; RBANS: Repeatable Battery for the Assessment of Neuropsychological Status. MoCA: Montreal Cognitive Assessment; Penn CNB: Penn Computerized Neurocognitive Battery. SCoRS: Schizophrenia Cognitive Rating Scale; CGI-CogS: Clinical Global Impression of Cognition in Schizophrenia; BRIEF: Brief Rating Inventory of Executive Function; CAI: Cognition Assessment Interview.

COGSTATE battery (Pietrzak et al., 2009). Computerized test batteries have an advantage of minimizing human error and implementation across settings reliably, though they may not be widely available.

Although objective measures of cognition using neuropsychological test batteries as discussed above are the standard practice, interview-based measures that tap into subjective assessment of cognition are useful in clinical practice. One such measure is SCoRS (Keefe et al., 2006), which has 20 items rated 1–4 covering all seven MCCB domains and administered to the patient and an informant. Scores from this instrument correlate well with objective measures of cognition as well as with real world functioning (Keefe et al., 2006). Other interview-based cognitive assessment measures include CAI and CGI-CogS (Ventura et al., 2008, 2013). While these assessment tools are easy to administer and practical, their validity, i.e. their relation to objective measures of cognitive function, continues to be studied.

Assessing Social Cognition

There are several approaches to assess social cognition (Table 1.2). A common test is the Penn Emotion Recognition Test which involves recognizing emotions in pictures (Gur et al., 2001). One objective measure, MSCEIT, a measure of emotion processing and management (Mayer et al., 2003), has now been added as a component of the MATRICS battery for schizophrenia, described earlier. Several tests are used to measure the Theory of Mind ability. One such test, The Awareness of Social Inferences Test (TASIT) assesses mentalizing processes depicted in videotaped interactions between adults, such as forming inferences about others' intentions and detecting white lies and sarcasm (McDonald et al., 2003). A common test used to assess context appraisal is the Social Cue Recognition Test (Corrigan & Green, 1993), which involves watching videotapes of two or three individuals interacting in low or high emotional situations, and answering true/false questions about the social cues displayed in these interactions.

Table 1.2 Domains of social cognitions and representative tests

Domain	Test	References
Emotion processing	Penn Computerized Neurocognitive Battery – Emotion recognition test	Kohler et al., 2003
	The awareness of Social Inference test (Part 1)	McDonald et al., 2003
	Mayer Saloway Cramer Emotional Intelligence Test (MSCEIT)	Mayer et al., 2003
Attributional bias	Attributional style questionnaire	Peterson et al., 1982
Theory of mind	The awareness of Social Inference test (Parts 2 and 3)	McDonald et al., 2003
	False belief stories	Frith & Corcoran 1996
	Hinting task	Corcoran et al., 1995
	Reading the Mind in the Eyes test	Baron-Cohen et al., 2001
Social perception	Social cue recognition test	Corrigan & Green 1993
Social knowledge	Situational features recognition test	Corrigan & Green 1993

Assessing Metacognitive Abilities

Metacognitive functions are difficult to measure since these assessments involve complexity of thought rather than concrete accuracy (Lysaker et al., 2014). Metacognitive capacity within narrative interviews can be assessed using the Metacognition Assessment Scale (Lysaker et al., 2007). Insight can be measured using several scales such as the Scale to assess Unawareness in Mental Disorders (SUMD; Amador et al., 1993) and the Beck Cognitive Insight Scale (BCIS; Peterson, Beck, & Keefe, 2004).

Assessing Functional Outcome

While assessment of cognitive function is important in determining the efficacy of cognitive enhancement approaches, it is also necessary to examine the implications of such changes to the real world functional outcomes. The key aspects of functioning include (a) role functioning in areas such as work, school, and independent living; (b) quality of life as measured by subjective sense of well-being and satisfaction; (c) functional capacity which indexes social competence or skill in the context of role-play or simulated tasks; and (d) rehabilitation success as measured by paid or competitive employment.

A widely used performance-based measure of functional capacity is the UCSD Performance-based Skills Assessment (UPSA) developed by Patterson et al. (2001). An abbreviated form, UPSA-brief is also available. Both are shown to be feasible and valid in clinical trial studies (Mausbach et al., 2007). Recently functional outcome assessment tools have been developed using virtual reality, such as the Virtual Reality Functional Capacity Assessment (VRFCAT; Ruse et al., 2014). Several tools to assess quality of life are available, such as the WHOQOL brief (Whoqol, 1998).

Neuroscience-based Measures

In recent years, there has been a recognized need to develop tests based on cognitive neuroscience constructs that may have better neural validity and may be translatable to experimental animal models. The Cognitive Neuroscience Treatment Research to Improve Cognition in Schizophrenia (CNTRICS) initiative grew out of this need (Carter & Barch, 2007). CNTRICS battery tests are yet to be tested in clinical trial settings, and their psychometric properties remain to be established.

1.7 Neural Mechanisms Underlying Cognitive Deficits in Schizophrenia

The brain mechanisms underlying non-social and social cognition is becoming increasingly clear with advances in measurement and neuroimaging technologies that allow for innovative methods for probing social and emotional information processing. The literature in this field is vast, and a detailed description of this vast literature is beyond the scope of this chapter.

Neural correlates of attention (Figure 1.7) are complex, and include three networks: *alertness* (maintaining awareness), *orientation* (focusing on new information from sensory input), and *attentional control* systems. Global processes of arousal and alertness are mediated by the activity of bottom-up neural circuits involving the ascending reticular activating system and the thalamus. A second aspect of attention, the Orienting Response

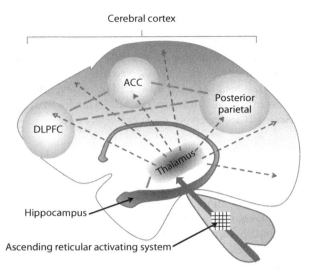

Figure 1.7 Brain regions involved in attention. Hatched regions (the ascending reticular activating system, the thalamus and thalamo-cortical projections) are important for bottom-up aspects of vigilance and general alertness, while blue regions represent key anterior and posterior nodes for top-down control of attention processes. DLPFC= dorsolateral prefrontal cortex; ACC= anterior cingulate cortex

(OR), also called *orienting reflex*, involves an organism's immediate response to a change in its environment. OR is related to activation of several dorsal and ventral brain regions including the prefrontal and parietal cortex, hippocampus, and the anterior cingulate. The *attentional control systems* include a wide range of brain regions including the anterior cingulate, the dorsolateral prefrontal cortex, and the posterior parietal cortex, which, respectively, form the anterior and posterior attentional systems.

The neural basis of working memory (Figure 1.8) has greatly been elucidated by lesion and neuroimaging studies. A large body of literature suggests that the prefrontal cortex, especially the Dorsolateral Prefrontal Cortex (DLPFC), is important for working memory, which is like scribbling on a mental scratch-pad. Patrícia Goldman-Rakic has shown that maintenance of working memory is mediated by recurrent excitation of glutamate containing neurons and regulated by dopamine and Gamma Amino Butyric Acid (GABA) neurons; persistent activation of these neurons allows maintenance of mental representations without external input (Goldman-Rakic & Selemon, 1997). There is some evidence that the left frontal cortex is involved in the maintenance of verbal working memory while the right prefrontal cortex is involved in spatial working memory. Working memory is not limited to the frontal cortex; a large number of other cortical brain regions are also involved. The anterior cingulate is involved in selective attention. Thus, while performing the Stroop task, the activity of the anterior cingulate is heightened (Carter, Botvinick, & Cohen, 1999).

The hippocampus, a structure shaped like a seahorse in the medial temporal lobe, is responsible for temporarily storing memories (like having a stack of manila folders on the top of your desk) which you can easily access that can be explicitly recalled (declarative memory). Consolidation of such memories occurs by transfer from the hippocampus to large areas of the cerebral cortex (like filing cabinets) in long-term memory (Squire & Zola-Morgan, 1991). Since brain regions such as the hippocampus mature during

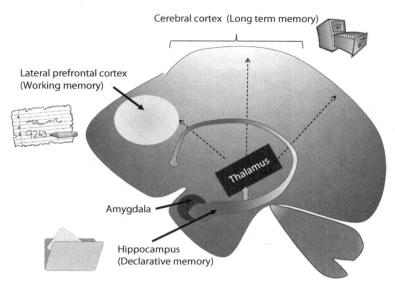

Figure 1.8 Brain regions involved in memory. The hippocampus mediates short term, declarative memory (like desktop files). The dorsolateral prefrontal cortex is a key node for working memories (which are like a mental scratch-pad). Amygdala is involved in emotional encoding of memories. Long-term consolidation of memories (like in a filing cabinet) results from transfer of memories from hippocampal stores to several cortical brain regions

the first few years of life, this form of memory is typically present after the first 2 years of life. Implicit memory is present from birth and probably involves several brain circuits including basal ganglia, limbic system, and perceptual cortical regions. The hippocampus also encodes emotional context from the amygdala. Thus, amygdala serves to "time-stamp" emotionally significant memories (think about how well you can remember what you were doing on September 11, 2001, though you may not so easily recall what you were doing on September 11, 2011).

Several brain circuits connecting frontal executive circuits to phylogenetically older medial–temporal and parietal regions of the brain are now known to support many of the social-cognitive abilities that are studied today (see Figure 1.9). Some of the earliest and most well-studied aspects of social cognition as they relate to neurobiology concern emotion appraisal (Phillips et al., 2003). The limbic structures of the brain have been consistently implicated in nearly every emotional task individuals have performed during functional brain imaging. The amygdala is perhaps the most studied brain region involved in emotion processing (Hamann et al., 2002), perception of emotion (Adolphs, Gosselin, & Buchanan, 2005), and regulation of emotion (Banks et al., 2007). The fusiform gyrus, an elongated medial temporal structure, is commonly activated when processing facial recognition and emotion processing (Kanwisher, McDermott, & Chun, 1997). Current models suggest that the sensory systems direct emotional data to both limbic and prefrontal circuits, and as the amygdala and other limbic structures become active, prefrontal areas of the brain (e.g. dorsolateral, medial, anterior cingulate and orbitofrontal prefrontal cortices) work to regulate the activity of these limbic regions to reduce arousal and lend interpretation (sometimes considered reappraisal) to emotional

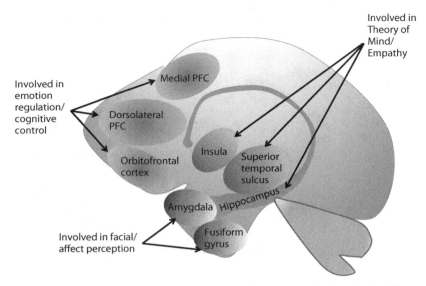

Figure 1.9 Brain regions involved in social cognition. PFC: Prefrontal Cortex. Those involved in affect perception are in red, those involved in cognitive control/affect regulation are in green, and those mediating theory of mind and empathy are in blue

experience (Perlman & Pelphrey, 2011). Perspective taking, which involves theory of mind discussed earlier, is mediated by activity of several brain regions including the temporoparietal junction (Saxe & Kanwisher, 2003). The superior temporal sulcus is involved in social perception (Allison, Puce, & McCarthy 2000) and the insula is among several brain regions involved in empathic processes (De Vignemont & Singer, 2006).

Neuroimaging studies have clearly implicated abnormalities in all the above circuits in schizophrenia. Impaired attention and executive functions have been related to alterations in the structural and functional integrity of the prefrontal, cingulate, inferior parietal, and superior temporal cortices, collectively termed the heteromodal association cortex (Pearlson et al., 1996). The language and thought disturbances in schizophrenia are related to disruptions in the structure and functioning of the superior temporal cortex and the planum temporale (Shenton et al., 1992). Deficits in declarative memory have been attributed to hippocampal volume reductions (Mathew et al., 2014). Impairments in cognitive control are related to aberrant functioning of the anterior cingulate (Kerns, Cohen, & MacDonald, 2005). Brain structural and functional alterations across a wide range of regions involved in social cognition functions such as emotion processing, empathy, and perspective taking have been found in schizophrenia (Fujiwara, Yassin, & Murai, 2015). Many of these observed alterations appear to be present in the premorbid phase of the illness, as evidenced by studies of familial high-risk relatives (Thermenos et al., 2013). Widespread gray matter alterations seem to progress during adolescence in individuals at clinical high risk (Cannon et al., 2015) as well as during the first several years of the illness (Thompson et al., 2001). All these observations underline the importance of targeting cognitive and brain changes in the early course of psychotic disorders, using neuroplasticity-based cognitive interventions, as will be discussed in the next chapters.

1.8 Summary

- Cognitive impairments are core aspects of schizophrenia. They are highly prevalent in the illness, prominent, present early in illness and persist through the course of the illness, and predict functional outcome.
- Cognitive deficits in schizophrenia are pervasive, and are seen across several domains, including speed of processing, memory (working memory, visual and verbal learning and memory), reasoning, and tact (social cognition).
- A wide range of objective approaches are available to assess cognitive function and real-world outcome before, during and after cognitive enhancement interventions.
- The brain mechanisms underlying social and nonsocial cognition are increasingly well understood, and implicate a distributed network of affected regions.

Chapter

2

The Brain That Builds Itself
The Phenomenon of Neuroplasticity

In this chapter, we will review a fundamental principle of the nervous system that underlies how cognitive enhancement approaches work. Plasticity refers to the property of the brain to change (be molded or sculpted) as a function of learning and experience (Figure 2.1). An understanding of neuroplasticity is important for efforts to develop neurobiologically informed therapeutic strategies for cognitive neurorehabilitation.

2.1 Neuroplasticity: A Historical Overview

For a long time, it was thought that once developed, the brain is immutable. Ramon Cajal, considered one of the founding fathers of modern neuroscience, thought that the adult brain is unlikely to change with experience (Ramon y Cajal, 1894). Cajal, however, later changed his mind and suggested that memories might be formed by strengthening the connections between existing neurons (Stahnisch & Nitsch, 2002).William James, a noted American psychologist, was among the first to suggest that the brain is not as immutable as previously thought. In his book *The Principles of Psychology*, James wrote, "Organic matter, especially nervous tissue, seems endowed with a very extraordinary degree of plasticity." (James, 1890). This view was ignored for several decades. An important milestone was the proposal by Canadian psychologist, Donald Hebb (Hebb, 1949) of an idea later referred to as "Hebbian learning." His view was that when two neurons repeatedly or persistently fire together, some changes take place in one or both cells such that the efficiency of neuronal activity is increased. The adage "neurons that fire together wire together" became the cornerstone of the concept of neuroplasticity, which refers to how the brain changes – organizes and reorganizes – in response to experience. While the brain shows plasticity throughout an individual's lifetime, its capacity for change may be higher at certain times than others; this led to the concept of Critical Periods, discussed later in this chapter.

2.2 Neuroplasticity Has Many Forms

Brain plasticity has been defined in a number of different ways (Figure 2.2). First, plasticity can be seen both at the level of the synapse, neuron, glia (cells in the brain that are not neurons and serve supportive functions) and neural network. *Synaptic plasticity* is the ability of a synapse (the junction between two neurons) to change in strength over time, perhaps due to modifications in synaptic potentials or receptors that transmit chemical signals. Modification of synaptic strength is mediated by a phenomenon whereby repeated signal transmission between two neurons leads to long-term potentiation (LTP)

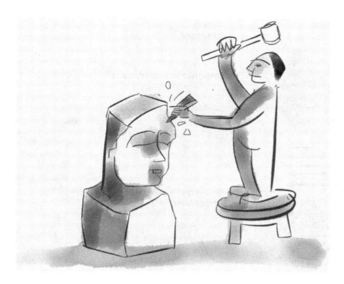

Figure 2.1 The concept of plasticity is similar to sculpting by experience

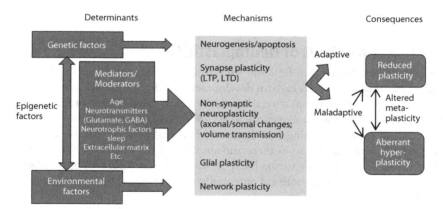

Figure 2.2 Types of neuroplasticity
Abbreviations: GABA: Gamma aminobutyric acid; LTP: Long-term potentiation; LTD: Long-term depression.

of neuronal activity (Lomo, 2003; see Figure 2.3). The opposite phenomenon, in which there is a net decrease in neural activity, is called long-term depression (LTD). By contrast, *non-synaptic plasticity* is a modification of the intrinsic excitability of the neuron, mediated through changes in structures such as the cell bodies, axons, and dendrites. This may happen through neuronal transmission that happens outside of synapses (e.g. by extracellular diffusion processes), using a process called volume transmission (Vizi, 1979), via glial changes, or even changes in blood vessels (Markham & Greenough, 2004). The production of new neurons (neurogenesis) as well as their programmed elimination (also called apoptosis) may also contribute to brain plasticity.

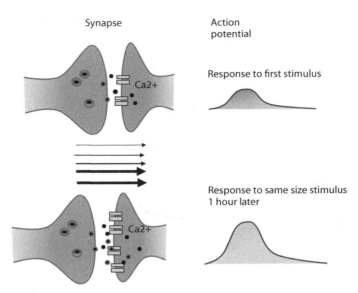

Figure 2.3 The phenomenon of long-term potentiation

2.3 Critical Windows of Neuroplasticity

Environment can shape brain function substantively across the lifespan. Plasticity is at its greatest during key epochs early in development (critical periods; Figure 2.4). Studies of critical periods in the visual cortex have shown that among other processes, maturation of specific gamma aminobutyric acid (GABA) circuits may determine the onset of certain critical periods. Timing and duration of critical periods may be modifiable by pharmacological manipulation of these and similar circuits (Takesian & Hensch, 2013). An understanding of such factors is likely to shed light on disorders of neuroplasticity such as schizophrenia, and motivate potentially novel treatment targets (Bitanihirwe & Woo, 2014).

Neuroplasticity may occur in two (not mutually exclusive) developmental contexts. Very early in development, experience and its resulting neuronal activity can shape neuronal response properties irrespective of an organism's attention to a stimulus. This process is called *experience–expectant neuroplasticity* (Hubel & Wiesel, 1959). For example, healthy infants need an expected visual input to develop the visual system, and infants with uncorrected congenital cataracts who fail to receive such input go on to develop permanent blindness. Such plasticity is often conceptualized to occur within a finite window, an early "critical period." Maladaptive experiences or insults to the developing brain during these critical periods can have lasting behavioral consequences. By contrast, *experience–dependent neuroplasticity* (Klintsova & Greenough, 1999) occurs *throughout* development. This process involves changes in neuronal activity in relation to experience, leading to lasting neural representations. Clearly, experience-dependent neuroplasticity is critically important as a mechanism of the therapeutic benefits of cognitive remediation (Nelson, 2000).

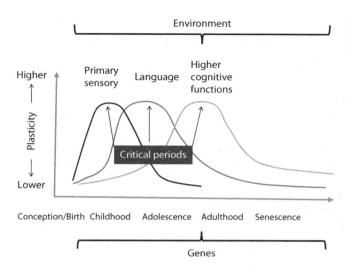

Figure 2.4 Critical windows of brain plasticity (for details see Nelson, 2000)

2.4 Neural Networks Are Constantly Remodified

In a landmark development in neuroscience, Michael Merzenich and colleagues showed in the 1980s that cortical maps can be modified with experience. The external and internal worlds of experience are point-by-point represented in maps on the cortex, so that a map for the hand lies adjacent to the maps of the face, the trunk, etc. This is called the Homunculus. Merzenich (Buonomano & Merzenich, 1998) showed that when the inputs to such maps are experimentally manipulated in monkeys, for example by cutting the median nerve, these maps change. Not surprisingly the relevant cortex no longer responds to stimulation of the fingers innervated by the median nerve; interestingly however, this area of brain begins to respond to stimulation of the adjacent fingers suggesting an expansion of the neighboring maps. This functional or network plasticity is a general principle across the nervous system.

Several lines off evidence support the concept of network plasticity with experience. Magnetoencephalographic studies in musicians have shown that cortical regions representing fingers show larger areas of activation upon stimulation. Interestingly the length of training correlated with the magnitude of activation (Elbert et al., 1995). London taxi drivers who have been driving for many years show larger hippocampi than comparison subjects (Maguire et al., 2000). Taken together, these observations suggest that a significant degree of functional plasticity continues throughout life in humans, a point of substantive importance to the field of cognitive enhancement. While the mechanisms underlying such plasticity remain to be fully elucidated, they clearly involve long-term experience-dependent changes in synaptic strengths in participating brain circuits.

2.5 Plasticity Cuts Both Ways

The brain can be reshaped in either *adaptive or maladaptive* ways. Aberrant plasticity can have profound impact on neuronal activity (Papa et al., 2014; Pirttimaki & Parri, 2013) and may be triggered in pathological conditions. Phantom limb sensations are a dramatic example of such maladaptive rewiring. Many individuals after amputation of a limb re-experience sensations from the missing limb when another part of the body such as the face is stimulated. Unwanted excessive plasticity has been implicated in addiction, PTSD, and depression, Alzheimer disease and Huntington disease (Oberman & Pascual-Leone, 2013; Pittenger, 2013).

The cardinal features of schizophrenia may also arise either from diminished plasticity or pathological excessive plasticity. For example, the core cognitive deficits in this illness are presumed to be related to learning impairments and diminished plasticity, and decreased cortical thickness (Keshavan et al., 2015), while psychotic symptoms are thought to be related to excessive "runaway" activity of hippocampal neurons (Tamminga, Stan, & Wagner, 2010). How can one understand excessive and decreased neuronal function and plasticity occurring together? In neurological disorders such as stroke, some symptoms such as paralysis are thought to result from failure of activity in some parts of the brain, while other symptoms such as hyperreflexia are thought to result from excessive unrestrained activity of other brain circuits in a pathological compensation. We have proposed – in an extension of this original model by neurologist Hughlings Jackson – a dysplasticity model in which hypoplastic brain circuits result in cognitive and deficit symptoms, and an aberrant hyperplastic response which might underlie psychosis and emotional dysregulation (Keshavan et al., 2015; Figure 2.5).

2.6 Nurture Can Shape Nature via Epigenetic Mechanisms

The ability of learning to shape the brain may also be related to epigenetic changes. Epigenetics refers to the activity of genes that can be altered by environmental experiences without changes in the underlying DNA sequence. In other words, while the genotype refers to the instruction manual we are born with, epigenetics refers to the question of which pages of the manual we open, depending on environmental inputs. The mechanisms of such epigenetic processes are increasingly better understood. Such mechanisms include DNA methylation (addition of a methyl group to a nucleotide which forms the

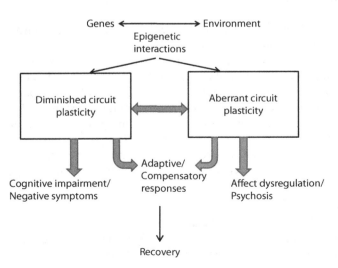

Figure 2.5 The dysplasticity model of schizophrenia (for details see Keshavan et al., 2015)

backbone of the DNA), and histone modification (modification of the proteins around which DNA is wrapped), both of which serve to modify gene function without altering the underlying DNA sequence. Further, non-coding RNA molecules (called microRNAs) can also alter gene expression. These microRNA molecules can "silence" the function of a gene by acting on messenger RNAs (molecules that carry information from genes to places in the cell where proteins are synthesized).

In a series of landmark experiments Michael Meaney at McGill University (Meaney, 2001) has shown that rat pups taken outside their maternal environments ("handled") for periods of time every day are more sensitive to stress than those that were licked and groomed affectionately by their mothers during a critical window of development. Pups which were reared by neglectful mothers also grew up to be fearful stressed-out neurotic rats. Even more interesting, they became neglectful mothers themselves as they gave birth to their offspring! This is an example of naturally occurring plasticity that transcends generations. Meaney and colleagues further showed that the deleterious effects of neglectful mothering in these rats can be reversed by adoption, early in life, to nurturing mother rats.

What underlies such changes in stress responsiveness that lasts a lifetime? Meaney and colleagues observed that the activity of the gene that produces corticosteroid receptors is turned up in rat pups that received the external maternal licking. Clearly, this is an epigenetic effect due to silencing of the gene coding for the corticosteroid receptor gene by methylation processes.

2.7 Experience-Dependent Plasticity Changes Throughout Life, Especially around Adolescence

The brain continues to develop from early intrauterine life through young adulthood. The initial steps in brain development include the birth of neurons (neurogenesis) in the dentate region of the hippocampus and periventricular brain regions, followed by neuronal proliferation and migration to their eventual location in the brain (see Figure 2.6). With increasing sensory and environmental input, synapses proliferate and connect with each other, leading to abundant neuronal connectivity reaching a plateau in early childhood.

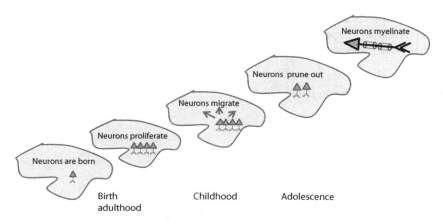

Figure 2.6 Phases of brain development

However, such abundance is not efficient for brain's operations. As we have discussed earlier, neuronal connections that are repeatedly used tend to persist and become strengthened, while those that are redundant and inefficient tend to be eliminated. This process of synaptic and axonal pruning begins in late childhood and continues through late adolescence (Huttenlocher, 1979). In parallel, axons that connect the functioning neurons expand in diameter and also develop myelin sheaths (like insulation around wires) around them which make them conduct faster and therefore more efficiently. This process of myelination, which begins in childhood, continues throughout adulthood (Keshavan et al., 2014).

Clearly, adolescence is a period where the processes of synaptic pruning and myelination are proceeding concurrently; it is no wonder that this is a critical period of development when cognitive functions such as executive functions, cognitive control, and abstract thinking develop. Such a maturation of cognitive functions is made possible by increasing efficiency in brain operations with elimination of redundant synapses, but at a cost: the reduced redundancy leads to diminishing brain plasticity. It is easy to see that a derailment of this process of brain maturation during adolescence, due to genetic or environmental factors, can result in disorders such as schizophrenia which typically begin during adolescence, as will be seen later in this chapter.

2.8 Several Factors Modify Brain Plasticity Throughout Life

While the brain continues to show some level of plasticity throughout life, its capacity to change is at its peak early in life, and gradually diminishes with age after young adulthood, as discussed above. However, there is an enormous variation between individuals in the degree, slope, and timing of plasticity; both genetic and environmental factors including lifestyle account for such variation (Oberman & Pascual-Leone, 2013).

Several other factors may alter brain plasticity (Box 2.1). Deep brain stimulation, stress, antidepressants, and exercise have been shown to increase adult neurogenesis in rodent models (Eisch et al., 2008). While promising, most research on this topic has been conducted on animal models. New techniques are being developed for *in vivo* visualization of neurogenesis in humans, such as the use of metabolic biomarkers to identify neural stem cells using proton magnetic resonance spectroscopy (Manganas et al., 2007). Further technical advances may allow for direct study of neurogenesis in human neuropsychiatric illness.

Sleep is another important mediator of brain plasticity. It has been known for a long time that certain types of memory such as procedural memory (like learning to play a

---

Box 2.1 Factors affecting brain plasticity

Age

Sleep

Exercise

Stress

Brain stimulation techniques

Drugs (such as antidepressants)

musical instrument) "stick" better if the learning is followed by a good overnight sleep (Wamsley et al., 2012). A recent hypothesis suggests that the extensive sensory inputs and learning experiences during waking hours leads to synaptic strengthening which results in synaptic fatigue, and sleep is restorative, serving to reset this imbalance (Tononi & Cirelli, 2014). An interesting type of oscillation during non-rapid eye movement (NREM) called sleep spindles are thought to play a role in synaptic changes and sleep-dependent memory consolidation (Fogel et al., 2012). Spindle oscillations induce LTP-like synaptic plasticity, and facilitate sleep-dependent memory consolidation (Rosanova & Ulrich, 2005). Moreover, a simultaneous EEG-fMRI study showed that the functional connectivity of the hippocampal formation with the neocortex was the strongest during stage-2 NREM sleep when spindles were present (Andrade et al., 2011).

2.9 Plasticity As Compensation

The idea that we have in-built mechanisms to overcome losses or deficits is not new. To paraphrase Ralph Waldo Emerson's 1841 essay "it is not only that there is a balancing gain for every loss but there is also a balancing loss for every gain ... compensation everywhere" (Emerson, 2000). Alfred Adler (Adler, 1927) viewed compensation as a critical defense mechanism for survival. There are several levels of compensation. At a behavioral level, in order to compensate for a deficit, one can: (a) voluntarily invest more time and effort in training or working harder; (b) overcome a deficit by developing a new skill or substituting it with a latent skill; (c) accommodate one's own expectations and/or priorities; and/or (d) adapt the environment to adjust the task demands to one's own performance (Dixon & Bäckman, 1992–1993). Compensation also occurs at neural levels. At a synaptic level, compensation may be related to dendritic changes such as increased arborization and density. Neural circuits may also undergo collateral sprouting and regeneration; compensatory reallocation of neural resources may also occur. While such brain adaptation may serve to overcome deficits, they come often with the cost of decreasing neural efficiency. Elucidating conditions where such compensatory processes work toward advantageous versus disadvantageous outcomes is an important topic for research.

Behavioral and neural compensation processes are not independent. Voluntary compensatory processes occur with full awareness of the deficits, but over time, these processes may become less effortful, and more automatic, as neural adaptations take place. Effortful and automatic processes may complement each other, and may either be simultaneous or sequential (Dixon et al., 2008).

2.10 Altered Brain Plasticity in Psychiatric Disorders

There is increasing evidence for alterations in neuroplasticity in major psychiatric disorders, such as schizophrenia and autism (Oberman & Pascual-Leone, 2013). The typical onset of psychotic symptoms and cognitive decline during adolescence, and the observations of pronounced gray matter reductions around the onset of this illness have led to the hypothesis that schizophrenia may be related to an exaggeration of the normative synaptic pruning processes around adolescence (Figure 2.7). This view, originally proposed by Irwin Feinberg (Feinberg, 1982–1983; Keshavan, Anderson, & Pettegrew, 1994), has received subsequent support by observations of dendritic loss and synapse reductions in post-mortem studies of this illness (Glantz & Lewis, 2000). Reduced synaptic redundancy may also be expected to lead to diminished brain plasticity which can account for the

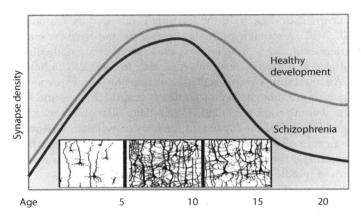

Figure 2.7 The developmental model of schizophrenia

cognitive deficits, negative symptoms, and functional disability central to this illness (Fett et al., 2011; Green et al., 2004; Sergi et al., 2007).

Evidence to support reduced cortical plasticity in schizophrenia comes from novel neuroimaging experiments that incorporate brain stimulation and electroencephalography (EEG). Transcranial magnetic stimulation (TMS) has been used to study *in vivo* cortical plasticity in schizophrenia. This method uses focal magnetic fields to penetrate the cranium. The resultant electric currents then depolarize the underlying cortex, thus inducing action potentials in targeted brain regions (Kobayashi & Pascual-Leone, 2003). The output of cortical activation (in this case motor cortex) is measured using electromyographic (EMG) recordings of hand muscle contractions. The most common method has been to compare motor-evoked potentials (MEP) and motor thresholds (MT) before and after repetitive brain stimulation – with repetitive TMS (rTMS) or transcranial direct current stimulation (tDCS) which uses direct currents to shift the resting membrane potentials of underlying neurons (Nitsche & Paulus, 2000). These techniques use synaptic plasticity-inducing protocols that result in cortical excitability changes mirroring LTP (high-frequency rTMS and anodal tDCS) or LTD (low-frequency rTMS and cathodal tDCS).

Compared to healthy controls, reduced LTD-like plasticity has been reported in schizophrenia patients by demonstrating lack of expected changes in MEP (reduction in amplitude) and MT (increase) as induced by low-frequency rTMS, delivered to the premotor (Oxley et al., 2004) and motor (Fitzgerald et al., 2004) cortices, as well as by cathodal tDCS delivered to the motor cortex (Hasan et al., 2012). Stimulus-specific plasticity paradigms using event-related potentials have also been used to quantify occipital (visual) and temporal (auditory) lobe LTP-like plasticity (Clapp et al., 2005a, 2005b). Here, repetitive high-frequency visual or auditory stimuli are used to produce a lasting facilitation of visual- or auditory-evoked potentials, respectively. Using this paradigm, researchers have demonstrated lesser facilitation of visual- (Cavus et al., 2012) and auditory- (Mears & Spencer, 2012) evoked potentials in schizophrenia patients as compared to healthy controls. Overall, these findings not only provide evidence for deficient cortical plasticity that represents both LTD- and LTP-like synaptic plasticity, but importantly, also link these deficits to impairments in cognitive functions such as learning and memory (Frantseva et al., 2008; Wamsley et al., 2012).

While reduced brain plasticity may explain the core cognitive deficits in schizophrenia, aberrant hyperplasticity (or hyperactivity) may underlie psychotic symptoms (Keshavan et al., 2015). This integrative pathophysiologic model (Figure 2.5) might explain the 'sequential emergence of negative symptoms and cognitive deficits followed by psychosis symptomatology in high-risk populations (Shah, 2017).

2.11 Plasticity Can Be Measured in the Human Brain

Until recently, it was only possible to study Brain plasticity by investigating LTP in *in vitro* cortical tissue. In recent years, techniques have been developed to non-invasively investigate LTP in healthy human tissue using TMS (rTMS) and EEG. Studies have shown that rTMS using paired associate stimulation can facilitate motor stimulation in healthy subjects but not in schizophrenia patients (Daskalakis et al., 2008). LTP-like plasticity can also be induced by repetitive sensory stimulation similar to the repetitive electrical stimulation used *in vitro*. Mears & Spencer (2012) have recently shown that event-related potentials (ERP) can be used to investigate brain plasticity after repetitive auditory stimulation at high frequency (10 Hz). While such stimulation resulted in enhanced plasticity and healthy controls, these effects were impaired in schizophrenia patients. Similarly, Cavus et al. (2012) used high-frequency visual stimulation (i.e. flickers at around 9 Hz) to potentiate visual-evoked potentials (VEPs) as a way to measure visual cortical plasticity. Again, such potentiation was seen in healthy controls but not in patients with schizophrenia.

Clearly, these methodological advances point to better and non-invasive ways to measure stimulus-specific brain plasticity in psychiatric illnesses many of which are disorders of neuroplasticity. These measures will also enable elucidating brain circuitry alterations and in disentangling effects of the disease from those of medications and psychosocial treatments. Finally, it may be possible to enhance neuroplasticity in a non-invasive manner, when used in conjunction with cognition remediation approaches.

2.12 Neuroplasticity Can Be Harnessed for Therapeutic (and Prophylactic) Gains

It is clear that observations of diminished as well as aberrant excessive plasticity motivate novel therapeutic as well as prophylactic therapeutic strategies in schizophrenia and the at-risk states for this illness. We herein provide examples of such emerging approaches (also see Chapter 7).

Cognitive training or cognitive enhancement is an evolving form of intervention that allows us to intentionally harness neuroplastic processes related to therapeutic learning, that targets the disabling cognitive deficits of schizophrenia (Keshavan et al., 2014). A recent meta-analysis suggested that cognitive training resulted in modest gains in cognition and socio-occupational functioning with mean effect sizes of 0.45 and 0.42, respectively (Wykes et al., 2011). Besides, the benefits of some of these interventions are likely to last beyond treatment cessation (Eack et al., 2010; Subramaniam et al., 2012; Wykes et al., 2003).

The underlying plastic changes with cognitive training have been explored by neuroimaging studies. Patients who received cognitive training showed less gray matter loss in the left parahippocampal and fusiform gyrus and greater gray matter increase in the left amygdala after 2 years of cognitive enhancement therapy, as compared to a non-specific supportive therapy (Figure 2.8) (Eack et al., 2010). Interestingly, patients with larger

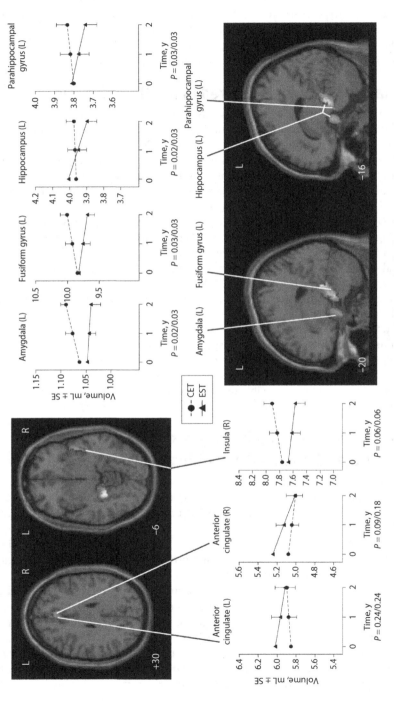

Figure 2.8 MRI data showing preservation of gray matter in key brain regions in schizophrenia following CET (Eack et al., 2010; with permission)

cortical thickness at baseline (higher cortical "reserve") improved faster (Keshavan et al., 2011). Computer-based cognitive training has been shown to normalize the task-based activation of the prefrontal regions during a reality-monitoring task (Subramaniam et al., 2012), emotional task-based neural activations in the postcentral gyrus (Hooker et al., 2012) and attention/executive task-based activations of the dorsolateral prefrontal cortex, anterior cingulate, and frontopolar cortex (Haut, Lim, & MacDonald, 2010). In addition, specific training of auditory discrimination and verbal memory and not a broadly administered cognitive training showed normalization of abnormally reduced sensory gating in schizophrenia patients as measured using magnetoencephalography (Popov et al., 2011). Diffusion tensor imaging (DTI) studies provide additional evidence by revealing normalization of the interhemispheric connectivity between the bilateral prefrontal cortexes via the corpus callosum in patients who received cognitive remediation (Penades et al., 2013). While structural and functional cortical plasticity changes have been demonstrated with cognitive training, one study also showed an increase in serum BDNF levels (Vinogradov et al., 2009).

2.13 Conclusion

Understanding the phenomenon of neuroplasticity is critically important to understand both, the core manifestations of schizophrenia (positive, negative, and cognitive symptoms) as well as the basis for cognitive enhancement approaches. In patients with schizophrenia as well as at-risk populations, plasticity alterations may involve both reduced plasticity in key brain systems serving cognitive functions and goal-directed behavior, and maladaptive excessive plasticity in neural systems underlying our ability to process and regulate emotions and make sense of the world. Preventive and therapeutic interventions with medications, neuromodulation, and psychosocial cognitive enhancement interventions may help reverse plasticity deficits as well as harness compensatory neuroplasticity in more adaptive channels. The increasing understanding of brain mechanisms underlying plasticity may suggest new ways of detecting preclinical disease, better biomarkers to guide treatment selection, and novel therapeutic targets. Several questions remain, however, as directions for future research. We still do not know what specific mechanisms of altered plasticity might contribute to schizophrenia, and whether they are primary rather than secondary to other pathophysiological processes. The gene–environment interactions that underlying such mechanisms need to be elucidated. We still need to know whether differences in plasticity capacities predict differential outcome trajectories. The best ways, pharmacological as well as psychosocial, to non-invasively harness plasticity in the service of prevention and early intervention need to be determined.

2.14 Summary

- The brain has a remarkable ability to change with experience, a phenomenon known as neuroplasticity.
- While the brain shows plasticity throughout an individual's lifetime, its capacity to change may be higher at certain times than others; which are known as critical periods.
- Plasticity can work in either *adaptive* or *maladaptive* ways. Both increased and decreased plasticity can cause emotional and behavioral difficulties, including cognitive impairments.

- Many psychiatric disorders such as schizophrenia may be related to alterations in brain plasticity. In schizophrenia, there may a diminished plasticity because of an excessive loss of, or impaired development of, synapses and other neural elements.
- Brain plasticity can be harnessed for therapeutic purposes by cognitive interventions, as well as pharmacological and brain stimulation approaches.

Cognitive Enhancement
Historical Overview and Principles

In this chapter, we provide a historical overview of cognitive enhancement approaches to psychiatric disorders, with an emphasis on schizophrenia and related disorders. The fundamental approaches, neural targets, and principles behind cognitive enhancement will be reviewed. This will be followed by a discussion of the factors that underlie successful outcomes with cognitive enhancement approaches at the patient level and at the level of the therapeutic setting,

3.1 Historical Overview

Clinical interest in "brain remediation" dates back to World War I when methods were developed to treat soldiers with war-related brain injuries. Recognition of cognitive impairments in schizophrenia dates back to the early part of the last century ever since Kraepelin described dementia praecox as an illness whose core manifestation is cognitive decline. However, the introduction of treatment for cognitive deficits was delayed by several decades; this may be traced back to at least three reasons. Cognitive impairments were attributed, during the first half of the last century, to the more firmly held psychodynamic theories of psychotic disorders; for example, Silvano Arieti, a psychoanalyst (1974) reasoned that concrete thinking in schizophrenia may be related to regression to earlier childhood levels of functioning. The second reason for slow progress in cognitive remediation efforts was the pessimism that resulted from the failure of initial cognitive treatment studies that had been conducted for brain injuries after World War II. Finally, therapeutic optimism in this field had to await basic science discoveries beginning in the 1960s motivating a theory-driven design of cognitive treatments, with an emphasis on harnessing neuroplasticity, the brain's inherent capacities for change in order to promote or restore adaptive cognitive and socio-affective processes (see Chapter 2).

It is instructive to trace the development of cognitive enhancement approaches in psychotic disorders over the past century (Figure 3.1). In the first half of the twentieth century, psychodynamic psychotherapy approaches were dominant. The beginning understanding of social and interpersonal factors in the pathogenesis of psychotic disorders led to the development of major role therapy, one of the first case management models (Hogarty, 1974). The important influence of family processes in schizophrenia subsequently led to family psychoeducation in the 1970s and 1980s (Anderson et al., 1980).

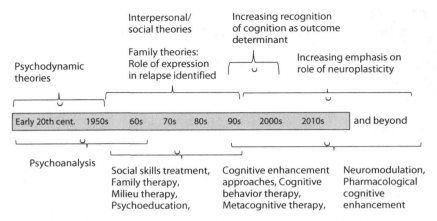

Figure 3.1 Evolution of psychosocial and cognitive enhancement treatments in schizophrenia

An approach to psychotherapy directed toward the unique aspects of schizophrenia, i.e. Personal Therapy, was developed in the 1990s (Hogarty, 2002) to address the chaotic early course of psychotic disorders and reduce relapse (see Chapter 5). However, the persistent cognitive symptoms in the illness which were relatively non-responsive to these interventions were noted to be key rate limiting factors toward recovery. At the same time, several studies began to demonstrate the important predictive role of cognitive impairment for functional outcome in schizophrenia summarized by Green (2000). Around this time, the emerging literature on the benefit of cognitive enhancement techniques focusing on basic cognitive processes in traumatic brain injury (Ben-Yishay & Prigatano, 1990) was inspiring optimism that similar approaches may work in schizophrenia. Social cognition was becoming a focus of interest around this time (Brothers, Ring, & Kling, 1990); Brenner and colleagues (1980) combined basic cognitive training with social perception training and this was subsequently adapted by Hogarty & Greenwald (2006) and Spaulding (1992). Hogarty and colleagues combined all of these insights to develop a manual for Cognitive Enhancement Therapy in the late 1990s and conducted intervention trials in schizophrenia patients (see Chapter 6). Keshavan & Hogarty (1999) around this time recognized the importance of brain developmental processes around adolescence for the emergence of social cognition and secondary socialization processes. They emphasized the role of a developmental impairment in schizophrenia leading to a pre-adolescent pattern of cognitive and social cognitive functioning in this illness. This led to a second, independent study of CET in early course schizophrenia patients (Eack et al., 2009, 2010). At the same time, many other groups were developing cognitive remediation interventions focused on attention, working memory, and executive functioning using a variety of paper-and-pencil, group-based, and computer-based approaches (e.g. Bell, Bryson, & Wexler, 2003; Silverstein et al., 2005; Wykes et al., 2007).

3.2 Definitions and Approaches to Cognitive Enhancement

The scientific literature is replete with terms such as cognitive enhancement, cognitive training, cognitive remediation, and cognitive rehabilitation which are used interchangeably and inconsistently. Cognitive remediation has been defined as "a behavioral

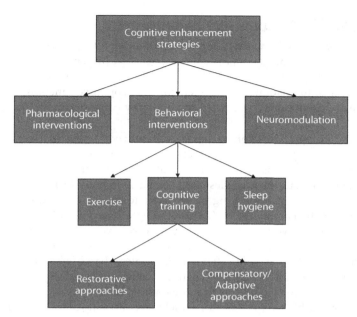

Figure 3.2 Taxonomy of cognitive enhancement approaches (for details, see Keshavan et al., 2014)

training-based intervention that aims to improve cognitive processes with the general aim of durability and generalization to community functioning" (Cognitive Remediation Expert Working Group, cited in Cella, Reeder, & Wykes, 2015).

We prefer to use the term cognitive enhancement both because it is less stigmatizing, is applicable to both healthy and ill populations, and because it provides a broad range of approaches to potentially improve cognitive functions. The terms "remediation" and "rehabilitation" imply the presence of a deficit, which most patients do experience, but this does not apply as well to situations where the goal is to improve upon functions that are within normal limits, but may be below what is expected. For example, some patients with schizophrenia or bipolar disorder exhibit cognitive performance that is within a normal range but far below their own potential. Individuals who are at high risk for psychosis prior to psychosis onset, may also benefit from cognitive enhancement (not necessarily remediation) as a way to build cognitive reserves that may protect against cognitive and functional decline. It is important to recognize that we herein use cognitive enhancement as a broad term for many different approaches (Figure 3.2) and that it is not synonymous with the specific approach of Cognitive Enhancement Therapy (Hogarty & Greenwald, 2006).

Cognitive enhancement approaches differ from cognitive behavioral therapy (CBT), which focuses more on the content (as opposed to the processes) of cognition and thought. However, this distinction of form versus content is blurred because the content of metacognitive strategies and schemas are highly important for cognitive enhancement. Cognitive enhancement also differs from other forms of broad educational and social interventions such as psychoeducation, social skills training, the 12-step program, or support groups. However, cognitive enhancement defined as above is typically embedded in a larger therapeutic context that makes use of therapist and participant expectancy, instillation of hope, and other important psychosocial ingredients.

3.3 Approaches to Cognitive Enhancement

There are three broad approaches to cognitive enhancement in general. First, the *remediation* of deficits in elementary processes of cognition by repeated *drill-and-practice*, either basic sensory processing or attention/executive functions with the expectation that this will generalize to restoration of higher, complex cognitive functions (Fisher et al., 2009). These approaches may be carried out either by computer programs or by paper and pencil.

Second, the *strategy-based* approaches seek to enhance cognitive functions by using one or more of "top-down" cognitive functions: (1) facilitating new and more efficient strategies for memory (e.g. using mnemonics), attention and information processing; and (2) enhancing metacognitive strategies (see Chapter 1) to boost learning. Metacognitive processes include (1) self-monitoring of performance which is essential for sustained learning (Tullis & Benjamin, 2011), (2) developing a repertoire of alternate strategies from which to choose while learning to function in novel situations, and (3) engagement in cognitive control to efficiently allocate attentional resources for cognitive tasks (Thiede, Anderson, & Therriault, 2003). Both strategy-based and drill-and-practice-based training are restorative forms of cognitive enhancement, designed to improve or restore cognitive functions to healthy or more optimal levels.

The third approach, *cognitive adaptation* includes enhancing cognitive performance by adapting the environment to place less demand on functions where deficits are observed (Velligan et al., 2000). These approaches, which involve modifications in the environment such as reminders, checklists, calendars, hygiene supplies, and pill boxes, etc., are designed to enhance adaptive function in the home or work setting. Such approaches can improve functioning; restoration of deficits in cognition may not be necessary for such benefits. On the other hand, it is possible that improvement in functional outcome itself may have a positive impact on cognition (Fredrick et al., 2015). *Compensatory cognitive training* developed by Elizabeth Twamley and colleagues is an approach that combines strategy-based and environmental adaptation approaches as applied to a wide range of real world situations. Controlled studies have shown that this intervention leads to improvements in cognition, psychopathology, functional capacity as well as quality of life (Twamley et al., 2012). There is evidence that this intervention may be helpful to patients with low cognitive performance and ability (Twamley, Burton, & Vella, 2011).

One way to remember the three approaches to cognitive rehabilitation (compensation, adaptation, and remediation) is to use the CAR acronym and metaphor. Imagine that the cognitive task is driving to a destination on time in slow traffic. You can (a) take a short-cut, an alternate route or alternative transportation, such as the train (compensation), (b) cancel or postpone your appointment, or simply relax and enjoy music while driving in the slow traffic (adaptation), or (c) increase your speed, or take a faster lane (remediation). Addressing the cognitive limitations in schizophrenia patients, whose core problem includes slow information processing, may require more than one approach.

3.4 Neural Targets for Cognitive Enhancement

As reviewed in Chapter 1, deficits in cognitive and emotional functions are highly prevalent in schizophrenia and related disorders, often predate the symptoms, and may predict functional outcomes (Liu et al., 2015). As reviewed in Chapter 1, alterations in neural circuitries supporting executive function, affect regulation, motivation, incentive salience, representations of self and other, and social perception underlie the cognitive and affective impairments in these disorders (Keshavan et al., 2014). Psychosocial interventions can potentially harness inherent plasticity processes throughout these relevant distributed neural systems (see Chapter 2) and presumably drive improvement in neural operations (Keshavan et al., 2014). Modification of macro-circuit neural function could have downstream effects on synaptic function at a micro-circuit level, including neurotransmitter and neurotrophic systems (McNab et al., 2009).

Cognitive interventions can work via "bottom-up" or "feed-forward" processes (such as perception and pre-attentive perceptual biasing) and/or "top-down" or "feedback" processes (e.g. attention, cognitive control, metacognitive appraisal) (Figure 3.3). Schizophrenia is characterized by cognitive impairments that range from impaired perceptual processes to inefficient prefrontal operations including working memory, episodic memory, and social cognition (Chapter 1). Impairments in sensory encoding (Javitt, 2009) may lead to degraded or "noisy" neural representations of sensory information being transmitted and thereby taxing working memory and attentional systems (Adcock et al., 2009). In affective disorders, impairments in attention, executive function, and processing speed are observed, associated with altered activity in fronto-parietal and limbic system networks associated with affect dysregulation (Brady et al., 2017), as well as abnormal biasing of attention to negative cognitions (Browning et al., 2010). These distinct and cross-cutting patterns of neural system dysfunction suggest that unique combinations of cognitive and socio-affective targets may be available for cognitive training across various psychiatric disorders. Inefficiencies or biases in prefrontal predictive and cognitive control operations may represent a fundamental or "common denominator" underlying a range of mental illnesses, resulting in disorder-specific or cross-diagnostic impairments or biases in perception, affect, and cognition (Keshavan et al., 2014). Such processes may represent promising targets for cognitive enhancement approaches, not

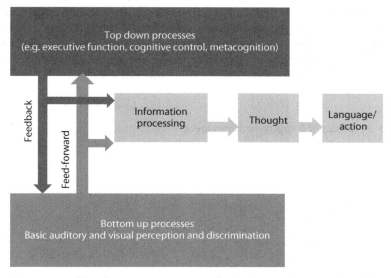

Figure 3.3 Bottom-up and Top-down cognitive processes (for details, see Keshavan et al., 2014)

only as a treatment, but also potentially as a preventive or pre-emptive intervention. However, it is to be kept in mind that no current assessment or intervention approaches address single neural system targets; changes in one brain system (e.g. attention) inevitably affect other systems (such as working memory and executive function).

3.5 Treatment-Related Principles That Underlie Success in Cognitive Enhancement Interventions

Several key principles (summarized in Box 3.1 by the acronym "TARGETS") that underlie therapeutic benefits of cognitive enhancement have to be considered while designing the intervention approaches. These are derived from the principles of neuroplasticity outlined earlier, as well as from literature in education and rehabilitation.

Targeted Interventions

As discussed earlier, cognitive enhancement approaches target a wide range of functions. These include basic constructs such as visual and auditory perception and attention, as well as higher order functions such as language and executive function, metacognitive strategies and social cognition. One approach is to start with simple, basic (bottom-up) sensory functioning, and gradually build strategies to improve higher cognitive functions (top-down mechanisms). Another approach is to target both sets of functions; currently it is unclear which of these approaches are better though there is some evidence that both are important (Nuechterlein, 2014; Wykes et al., 2011). The available training programs widely vary in this regard, with Posit-science (now called BrainHQ) taking the former approach, while others such as Cogpack (see Chapter 5) take the latter approach.

Adaptive and Progressive

Success with cognitive training is more likely when the tasks are neither overly difficult with high demand leading to frustration nor too easy making them less engaging. Activities that automatically adapt to learner performance keeping the difficulty level slightly but not overly challenging increase a sense of self-efficacy, and are therefore more likely to succeed. Learning also tends to be better when it is progressive. All new learning requires a foundation of prior learning. For example, one needs arithmetic before learning algebra and one needs algebra before learning trigonometry!

Box 3.1 Principles of cognitive enhancement

Targeted interventions

Adaptive and progressive

Repetition and practice

Generalization of learning

Engagement and motivation

Tailoring interventions to the individual

Strategy training and scalability

Repetition and Practice

It is widely believed by teachers and clinicians that the most effective way to enhance learning and skill building is to practice again and again. Repetition clearly increases the amount retained and the length of retention of learnt information (see Figure 3.4). When we learn something for the first time, we forget exponentially, as seen in the forgetting curve, attributed originally to the German Psychologist Hermann Ebbinghaus. When we relearn or review the information, the amount of information learnt peaks again, and the next time less if forgotten, or more is retained. This phenomenon provides a solid basis for the importance of repetition and practice in cognitive enhancement and education generally. However, studies often challenge this conventional wisdom; massed (or repetitive) practice may produce the illusion of being more skilled but does not necessarily lead to mastery or generalization. This is because the learning curve (dashed line in the figure) tends to be non-linear, with diminishing returns with each practice, and a plateau is reached after several repetitions.

Learning tends to "stick" better and is deeper when it is effortful (Brown, Roediger, & Mcdaniel, 2017). One approach to enhance learning is retrieval practice i.e. recalling concepts or facts from memory, or being quizzed about what is learned. There is evidence that *spaced practice* is more effective in retention of material than rapid-fire practice (Cepeda et al., 2006). Learning is more effective when presentations of information are separated in time than when offered back-to-back in immediate succession. This may be related to the need for consolidation of learned to material into long-term memories which may take several days and may involve process of rehearsal and retrieval. Such consolidation may also benefit from adequate sleep between learning and recall (Tamminen et al., 2010; also see Chapter 2).

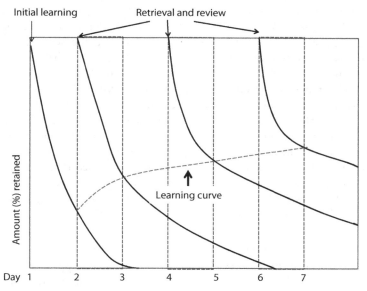

Figure 3.4 Forgetting curves with learning, and the effects of repetition and practice. Originally attributed to the German psychologist Hermann Ebbinghaus. Solid lines represent forgetting, and dashed line represents the learning curve

There is also evidence from educational literature that *interleaved practice* may be more effective than massed practice (Carpenter & Mueller, 2013). A conventional approach in teaching is to use "blocked practice" wherein repeated exposures are given to one concept at a time, followed by the next (e.g. AAA, BBB, CCC). By contrast, interleaved practice involves presentation of a mixture of all of the concepts presented together or in sequence in unpredictable order (e.g. ABC, CBA, BAC). An example is to learn mathematics, language, and science in interleaved classes throughout the week, in contrast with learning mathematics for one semester, Spanish for the next, etc. Several studies suggest that interleaving produces better learning than blocked practice in mathematics, category learning, and vocabulary learning (Kornell & Bjork, 2008; Mayfield & Chase, 2002). It has been suggested that interleaving helps the individuals make better discriminations between concepts that are otherwise easily confused.

Two additional concepts are important to understand the role of repetition and practice in cognitive training: scaffolding and errorless learning. *Scaffolding*, a concept derived from scaffolds which support a building's construction, is a framework for a learner to perform within the limits of his/her capacity. As the building develops, the scaffold is removed; likewise, as the individual learns, the scaffolds (like training wheels) are faded, so that more autonomy is transferred to the learner from the trainer. Scaffolding is used at the macro-level for treatment as a whole, with a larger amount of structure initially, with the goal of transferring the responsibility to the trainees. At a micro-level (e.g. within individual sessions), individual tasks are scaffolded using techniques of initial explicit instruction of key strategic elements of performance. Other learning principles include shaping (modelling accurate performance by trainer), operant conditioning (accurate performance is reinforced, and inaccurate performance is ignored) and fading of visual or auditory cues that assist performance. Errorless learning refers to strategies that minimize errors and maximize success (as in rote learning) so that the individual can capitalize on implicit memory and does not have to rely on explicit memory retrieval for performance (Baddeley & Wilson, 1994). This helps individuals with schizophrenia who have difficulties distinguishing between correct and incorrect memory. In this approach, a cognitive task is broken down into its components; training is then carried out stepwise, starting with the simplest components which are overlearned. More elements are then added with repetitive practice and positive reinforcements. Using this approach, Kern et al. (1996) have shown significant improvements in performance on the Wisconsin Card Sorting Test. However, the generalization of task-learning using this approach for other cognitive domains and community functioning is uncertain. Some conceptualizations of errorless learning were also based on the premise that schizophrenia patients cannot learn from their mistakes, which of course is not based in evidence and can be infantilizing to patients. We continually observe that patients with schizophrenia can and do learn from their own mistakes, and this is an important source of growth, as it is for many individuals with and without neuropsychiatric conditions.

Generalization of Learning

An important aspect of the success of cognitive enhancement approaches is the ability to generalize or transfer learning from tasks in which the training was carried out to situations demanding similar, though not identical situations. There are two types of transfer of learning: first, learning by extensive practice successfully transfers when there is a high similarity between the learning situation and another situation where implementation is needed. This "near transfer" characterizes many neurocognitive training approaches which show significant within-domain transfer of learning between similar tasks (Krabbendam & Aleman, 2003). By contrast, transfer to cognitive domains in which training had not occurred, or to non-cognitive tasks of everyday life (also called "far transfer, or cross-domain transfer") is not often seen in cognitive training studies. For such "far transfer" to occur, several factors appear important: (a) attention and other cognitive abilities; (b) metacognitive processing, and (c) domain-specific knowledge (Wykes & Reeder, 2005). For example, transfer of learning in declarative memory from a learning situation (e.g. remembering word lists) to actual real-world performance in a shopping mall will require (a) the ability to sustain attention and not be distracted while shopping, (b) an ability to categorize the items to remember better, e.g. vegetable, toiletries, and dairy, and (c) general shopping knowledge, e.g. where to look for the store and the needed items, and how to ask when one doesn't know.

Two key elements of cognitive training help in transfer of learning. First, generalization requires cognitive schemas (e.g. remembering the mnemonics or chunking strategies) to be retrieved from long-term memory that address similar solutions to the task trained in. The broader the schemas of initial learning, the more likely it is that connections are made between already learned and novel situations where transfer would happen (Cooper & Sweller, 1987). Second, transfer is more likely where the initial task learning is at a deeper, more abstract level than simply concrete learning (Greeno, 1989). These capacities underlying transfer of knowledge are likely to be impaired in schizophrenia both because of the deficits in declarative memory as well as the difficulties in the executive functions of categorizing and organizing information characteristic of this illness (see Chapter 1).

Engagement and Motivation

As stated earlier, motivation is a key factor in engagement and maintenance of effort in cognitive enhancement approaches. Programs that include motivational enhancements are therefore more likely to benefit from treatments. Users of computer training exercises tend to like visually appealing and game such as experiences, pleasing and rewarding sound experiences. Tasks that are interesting and varied also tend to be more engaging.

Patients with schizophrenia and related disorders are significantly impaired in motivation. Motivation may be related to external rewards such as money or prizes (*extrinsic motivation*) or to intrinsic factors (*intrinsic motivation*) associated with the task itself. Intrinsic motivation tends to lead to long-lasting enhancement of learning while extrinsic motivation's effects are faster though short-lasting (Ryan & Deci, 2000). Intrinsic motivation is increased when we (a) think we are competent at a given task (self-efficacy), (b) expect to experience success and pleasure (expectancy-value), and (c) have the ability and freedom to engage in the task (autonomy; Deci & Ryan, 1987). It is possible to enhance intrinsic motivation in cognitive enhancement settings using these principles (Choi & Medalia, 2010; Medalia & Saperstein, 2013).

Schizophrenia patients have significant impairments in motivation because of several reasons, including negative and persistent positive symptoms, depression, and low self-esteem. There are opportunity costs involved with having a chronic illness, as well as having impaired foresight causing difficulties in planning long term (Eack & Keshavan,

2008). All of these factors therefore need to be addressed early in stabilization of the schizophrenia illness (see Chapter 4) for cognitive enhancement efforts to succeed.

Tailoring Interventions to the Individual

Transfer (or generalization) of learning is more likely to happen during the use of activities of daily life especially of those that are personally meaningful to the individual, and to his or her life situation and goals (school, work, or relationships). Developing an individualized therapeutic plan in which personally relevant goals are identified and connected to the computer training strategies would be particularly helpful.

Patients with psychotic disorders vary considerably in their cognitive style, and this can have an impact on their response to cognitive treatments. Hogarty et al. (2004) have described three cognitive styles: disorganized, inflexible, and impoverished styles (also see Chapter 8). These categories roughly correspond to clusters derived from previous studies of heterogeneity in schizophrenia (Andreasen et al., 1990; Buchanan & Carpenter, 1994; Liddle, 1987). Briefly, patients in the *impoverished* group manifest predominantly negative symptoms; the *disorganized* cluster predominantly is characterized by disorganized thinking and *the reality distortion* cluster is characterized by delusions and hallucinations. There is a body of literature supporting somewhat distinct neuropsychological deficits across these clusters; subjects with the impoverished style are characterized by lack of relational schema and have to rely on effortful processing to retrieve stores of social cues. These patients tend to have flat affect, impaired planning, and initiation of behaviors and executive functioning suggesting deficits in the functioning of the dorsolateral prefrontal cortex and the dorsal stratum, though this aspect of literature is far from clear-cut (Chua et al., 1997). Patients with the disorganized style of thinking are characterized by impaired inhibition and affect dysregulation. These patients may show inattentiveness, derailment of speech, and inappropriate affect. This constellation of symptoms may be related to impaired orbitofrontal and medial and superior temporal cortical functions and show difficulties in attention and categorizing memory stores. Finally, patients with the rigid or inflexible style have impairments in developing alternative responses to the social situations because of a restricted repertoire of cognitive schema.

These cognitive styles are dimensional and not easily separable into categories; most patients may share characteristics of the different styles, although a single style is often predominant. Each individual needs to be carefully assessed for his/her unique styles at the beginning, and treatment strategies need to be adapted to these styles, as will be discussed later in this volume (see Chapters 6 and 8).

Strategy Training

Strategy training is the process of helping patients to develop explicitly planned strategies for solving cognitive problems and generalizing these to everyday life. Meta-analyses suggest that drill-and-practice training alone may not be as effective as those approaches that incorporate an element of strategic training in addition to repetition (Wykes et al., 2011). The premise is that repetition alone may only support improvement on the specific task, but if patients can develop strategies for enhancing performance beyond repetition (e.g. use of mnemonics, chunking), such strategies can be practiced in training and taken to the outside world for generalization. In doing so, the clinician helps the patient become more strategic in their problem-solving generally. By implementing strategy training, patients not only learn how to improve their performance on cognitive training tasks, but also develop generalizable strategies for solving challenging cognitive and other life problems outside the cognitive training context.

Scalability

Cognitive impairments are seen across a wide range of psychiatric disorders. The differences between cognitive impairments across the psychotic spectrum disorders (schizophrenia, schizoaffective disorder, psychotic bipolar disorder, and psychotic major depression) are more quantitative rather than qualitative (Hill et al., 2013). Other neuropsychiatric disorders may have a preponderance of one or other cognitive domain being affected, such as attention in attention deficit disorders, and social cognition in autism spectrum disorders. Many cognitive enhancement approaches used in schizophrenia such as CET and SCIT (see Chapter 6) can therefore be scaled up to other disorders, with the appropriate emphasis on disorder-specific cognitive issues.

3.6 Patient-Level Factors Associated with Success in Cognitive Enhancement Approaches

Table 3.1 lists the factors associated with a favorable outcome with cognitive enhancement, including those related to the nature of the treatment (dose, duration, and the design issues outlined in Section 3.4), patient-related factors, and factors that pertain to the therapeutic setting. These issues are also further discussed in Chapter 8.

Baseline Cognitive Function

Several studies have investigated whether baseline cognitive function may have a predictive value for response to cognitive enhancement interventions. Vita et al. (2013) found in a study of 56 patients with schizophrenia that baseline cognitive function, in particular executive functions and verbal memory, was predictive of cognitive improvement after a 6-month intervention. Additionally, they showed that lower antipsychotic intake and stability from specific symptoms at baseline were also associated with better cognitive normalization. In a recent large study, Lindenmayer et al. (2017) examined neurocognitive, demographic, and psychopathological predictors of cognitive remediation in 137 patients with serious mental illness. They observed that younger age, higher education, and lower levels of negative and disorganized symptoms were predictive of better cognitive improvement.

Table 3.1 Factors related to therapeutic success in cognitive enhancement interventions

Treatment-related factors	Patient-related factors	Factors related to the therapeutic setting
Treatment dose	Age	Therapeutic alliance
Treatment duration	Severity of psychopathology	Supported employment
Approach to intervention	Baseline cognitive function	Supported education
Integration with other elements of treatment	Genetic factors	Housing issues
	Growth mindset	
	Baseline brain "reserve"	

While traditional neuropsychological testing conducted once prior to intervention may have moderate predictive value, repeated testing to determine change with training may provide information on the learning potential of the individual and may have additional predictive value (Raffard et al., 2009). Relatively little research has been conducted to examine this possibility.

Genetic and Biological Predictors of Response

Cognitive functioning is significantly associated with the genetic risk for schizophrenia, and there is considerable heterogeneity in the degree of cognitive impairment across psychotic disorders. For these reasons, it has been suggested that genetic risk for this illness may predict therapeutic response to cognitive remediation. Catechol-O-Methyl Transferase (COMT) gene polymorphisms have been known to influence cognitive function in schizophrenia by their modulation of prefrontal dopaminergic activity. Bosia et al. (2007) observed that Met/Met alleles of the COMT gene were favorably associated with beneficial response to cognitive remediation. However, Greenwood et al. (2011) failed to see such an association. In a larger study, Lindenmayer et al. (2015) recently examined the association of COMT polymorphisms on therapeutic response to computerized cognitive remediation in 145 patients with schizophrenia or schizoaffective disorder. They observed that Met/Met and Met/Val groups, which have lower activity on prefrontal dopaminergic metabolism, are associated with greater improvements in the domains of verbal and visual learning and attention/vigilance. Given the potential role of a large number of genes in schizophrenia it would be important to examine multiple gene (polygenic) contributions to the therapeutic response to cognitive remediation. Indeed, a recent study showed that higher polygene risk factor scores were associated with a less prominent structural impact of aerobic exercise combined with cognitive remediation on the hippocampus (i.e. less volume increases) in patients with schizophrenia (Papiol et al., 2017). Clearly, larger studies are needed, given the relatively small amount of variation in cognitive function that is accounted for by genetic factors.

Neurobiological factors such as baseline neuroplasticity, brain structure, and function ("brain reserve") may potentially influence response to cognitive enhancement, and are further discussed in Chapter 8.

Growth Mindset

In recent years, work by Carol Dweck on the growth mindset (Dweck, 2015) has received a considerable amount of attention. This is based on the simple notion that one's intellectual capability is not "fixed" but to a large extent is under one's own control. In an early experiment in New York City Junior High School, Dweck ran a workshop where half the group received a presentation that intelligence was largely under one's own control ("growth" mindset) and the other half were taught that their intellectual capacities were set by the natural talents they were born with ("fixed" mindset). The former group went on to become higher achievers than the latter group. Individuals who aim at performance goals to validate their abilities tend to avoid difficult tasks, while those who aim at learning goals to acquire new knowledge or skills tend to work harder and pick increasing challenges. In another study, Dweck found that students who were praised for their smarts picked easier puzzles than those who were praised for their effort. Children with a growth mindset may even overcome the deleterious effects of poverty on achievement (Claro, Paunesku, & Dweck, 2016). These studies point to the important principle that beyond innate abilities, a growth mindset and discipline may underlie success in learning endeavors.

Insight

An important characteristic of patients that may impact on therapeutic response to cognitive enhancement interventions is their level of insight. There are two kinds of insight: clinical insight which refers to the awareness of, and causal attributions toward symptoms, and the appreciation of need for treatment; and cognitive insight which refers to the metacognitive processes of reflecting on one's own thought processes (self-reflectiveness) and the willingness to re-evaluate beliefs (self-certainty). A common instrument for measuring cognitive insight is the Beck Cognitive Insight Scale (BCIS). Benoit and colleagues (2016) recently examined the predictive value of cognitive insight prior to cognitive remediation in 20 patients with schizophrenia. They found that lower cognitive certainty, which reflects higher willingness to correct cognitive errors, was associated with larger improvements in cognition. While the results of this small study need to be replicated, this measure may be of clinical value given ease of implementation in routine clinical settings.

3.7 Therapeutic Context of Cognitive Enhancement Approaches: Role of the Rehabilitation Setting

As we have discussed earlier, the success of cognitive enhancement methods is likely to be dependent on the overall psychiatric rehabilitation framework in which it is implemented. It is therefore useful to briefly review the concepts that underlie rehabilitation. While cognitive enhancement techniques increase the needed skills for functioning, rehabilitation provides the needed support and creates opportunities.

Therapeutic Alliance

One of the factors that may mediate therapeutic benefits with cognitive remediation is the quality of therapeutic alliance. Vyv Huddy (Huddy et al., 2012) examined the relationship between therapeutic alliance and outcomes with going to remediation in 49 individuals with schizophrenia. Participants who rated the alliance favorably stayed in treatment longer and reported better improvements in their main complaints but the memory performance per se did not differ. This suggests that therapeutic alliance is important for client satisfaction during treatment. In a subsequent report (Cella & Wykes, 2017) however, this research group reported that the therapeutic alliance was associated significantly with improvements in functioning as well.

Housing

Traditional housing models in the 1980s and 1990s assumed that people with serious mental disorders required constant supervision which was best provided by being housed together, in apartments owned by the mental health system and participation in the mental health treatment being a requirement. The advent of assertive community treatment (ACT) from the early 1980s led to an increasing trend for helping people to leave the hospital and live outside in the community with comprehensive services 24/7 to help people learn independent living skills and managing crisis. The success of these ACT programs and the consequent move away from the previous paternalistic psychiatric practice led to a set of principles called *supported housing*. This approach involves normalized permanent housing, assurance of privacy and location in communities of client choice along with individual and flexible support. This "housing first" model integrates ACT intensive case management, shared decision making and housing assistance. There is evidence that seriously mentally ill patients can maintain independent housing with adequate psychosocial support (Mueser et al., 2013). Contrary to previous concerns there is no evidence that such a process leads to negative consequences.

Individualized Placement and Support

Across the United States less than 15% of seriously mentally ill patients hold competitive employment. A major goal in psychiatric rehabilitation has therefore been to increase employment opportunities for people with serious mental illness. The traditional model of vocational rehabilitation has been to "train and place" i.e. with pre-employment assessment and offering preparatory experiences, transitional employment, and skills training before placement in competitive employment.

The focus of vocational rehabilitation began to change in the late 1980s, based on experience from the field of developmental disabilities, to a "place and train" model, a concept which came to be known as *supported employment*. Evidence-based approaches to supported employment focus on the following principles: (a) providing services to anyone who seeks employment regardless of symptoms, work history, or intellectual ability; (b) based on patient preference and choices; (c) involve rapid job searches; and (d) seeking competitive employment at or more than minimum wage, supervised by employers rather than by rehabilitation programs, competitively paid rather than sheltered or volunteer jobs. Rehabilitation and mental health treatments are integrated such that employment specialists closely interface with the mental health teams including case management and ACT staff. Individualized benefits counseling is also provided as needed. Several pragmatic clinical trials have shown that supported employment approaches lead to higher rates of employment, greater earnings, longer retention in jobs, and better work satisfaction (Bond & Drake, 2014).

3.8 Summary

- Cognitive enhancement interventions have developed over the last century progressively in parallel to our increasing understanding of the core cognitive dysfunctions in schizophrenia and related disorders.
- Cognitive rehabilitation involves restoration of cognitive deficits, use of strategy/ compensation approaches, and adaptation strategies to minimize demand on impaired functions. All these approaches are valuable in improving functioning in people with serious mental illness.
- Principles of cognitive enhancement include targeted, adaptive, progressive, strategic, and repeated practice, generalization to real-world functioning, engaging/ motivationally enhancing, tailored to the person's cognitive style, and scalable across diagnoses.
- Patient level factors such as cognition, insight, and brain "reserve"; therapeutic factors such as treatment alliance and rehabilitation setting are important for the success of cognitive enhancement approaches.

Getting Ready for Cognitive Enhancement
Patient Engagement, Stabilization, and Integration

Our experience over the past two decades has been that success in cognitive rehabilitation is critically dependent on optimum care in the early phase of psychotic disorders. This involves arriving at an appropriate diagnosis and developing an integrated, phase-specific plan for management of symptoms, functional impairment as well as the vulnerability to the illness. An individualized approach to therapy needs to integrate many key principles of evidence-based psychotherapy in chronic psychotic illness. These include psychoeducation, providing psychosocial and material support, managing stress, and addressing functional limitations (Keshavan & Eack, 2014). Table 4.1 lists these key principles, which we will outline in some detail. We refer the readers to Hogarty's excellent monograph on personal therapy (PT) which embodies these key disorder-relevant principles (Hogarty, 2002). While Hogarty organizes these theoretic goals in sequential phases, these phases are by no means clearly distinct. The specific components of the interventions will have to be tailored to the individual patient's phase of illness and recovery, specific deficits and/or domains to be targeted in therapy. A brief account, provided below, of the current state of understanding of the nature of psychotic disorders will place such a therapeutic approach in perspective. Subsequently, the basic components for supporting stabilization, readiness for cognitive enhancement, and functional recovery are discussed.

Table 4.1 Key principles of psychotherapy in the early course of schizophrenia (Hogarty, 2002)

	Basic	Intermediate	Advanced
Psychoeducation	Learning about illness, symptoms, treatments, and general approaches to address them	Learning one's own illness triggers (early warning signs) and coping strategies	Learning about nature of disability, and one's own functional limitations and strengths
Coping with stress	Awareness of general triggers of stress response; family, using therapists, and medications for stress relief; learning breathing and relaxation	Awareness of individualized cues of distress, and adaptive and maladaptive responses; individualized strategies to avoid and address stress; guided imagery	Developing strategies to address stress in unscripted inter-personal and vocational settings; criticism management
Resumption of functionality	Focus on self-care (nutrition, hygiene), resumption of recreational activities; developing a routine	Beginning participation in simple household tasks; set occupational/educational goals	Adjustment to disability; return to work or school; develop social skills to function in educational/vocational settings

4.1 Nature of Psychotic Disorders

Psychosis refers to a loss of contact with reality that occurs in several serious and common psychiatric disorders. It manifests most frequently as hallucinations, which are sensory experiences (such as hearing voices) in the absence of actual stimuli, and delusions, which are false beliefs (such as being persecuted, or having special powers) that are not shared by friends and family or supported by evidence. Disorganized thinking is also common, as are difficulties with social interactions and day-to-day functioning.

The diagnosis of psychotic disorders, as per the Diagnostic and Statistical Manual version 5 (American Psychiatric Association, 2013), is based on clinical features, with no input from laboratory-based biomarkers. Clinical features of psychotic disorders include *positive* symptoms (experiences or beliefs that should not be normally present) such as hallucinations, delusions, and disorganized speech and behavior; *negative* symptoms (loss of abilities that should normally be present) such as social withdrawal, lack of motivation, and impairments in *cognitive* abilities such as memory, attention, and problem-solving. For schizophrenia, the most serious of the psychotic disorders, two or more of the following symptoms should be present, including at least one from the first three, for at least 1 month: delusions, hallucinations, disorganized speech, grossly disorganized behavior, and negative symptoms (criterion set A). In addition, the illness must result in significant functional impairment (criterion B), persist for at least 6 months (criterion C), and should not be secondary to another psychotic disorder (criterion D) or another medical condition or substance abuse (criterion E).

Several other psychotic disorders need to be distinguished from schizophrenia. First, patients need to be assessed to rule out secondary psychoses caused by medical illness or substance abuse. Schizophreniform disorder is a term used for a clinical picture that resembles schizophrenia, but with a duration of less than 6 months. Those with psychotic symptoms of less than a month's duration are termed brief psychotic disorders. Schizoaffective disorder is characterized not only by similar positive and negative symptoms as in criterion set A, but also has an overlapping mood syndrome during a substantive portion of the overall illness and requires non-affective psychotic symptoms for at least 2 weeks. Psychotic bipolar disorder and psychotic major depressive disorder are characterized by the psychotic symptoms being confined to manic or depressive episodes. Delusional disorders are associated with prominent, well organized delusions, infrequent or no hallucinations, less thought disorder or functional impairment and well-preserved affect. Patients with psychotic symptoms that do not fit into any of the above categories are grouped under the category "psychosis not otherwise specified."

While positive and negative symptoms are the more obvious and striking symptoms of schizophrenia, cognitive symptoms have emerged as a crucial symptom domain. It is now believed that cognitive deficits account for most of the morbidity and functional decline seen in this illness, though they still do not constitute a requirement for the diagnosis in the DSM classification system. Cognitive symptoms tend to be stable over the lifespan, though their severity may vary at different phases of the disorder (see Chapter 1).

Schizophrenia and affective psychoses typically manifest in adolescence (Figure 4.1). Many individuals have premorbid cognitive or affective dysfunctions that date back to childhood (the premorbid phase), and a substantive proportion show subtle psychosis-like symptoms, personality changes and functional declines that precede the first psychotic episode by weeks, months, or years (the prodromal phase). The subsequent course

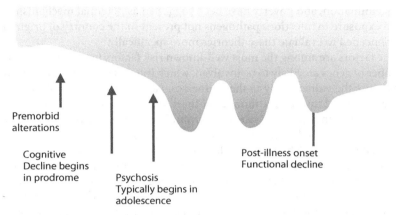

Premorbid
alterations

Cognitive
Decline begins
in prodrome

Psychosis
Typically begins in
adolescence

Post-illness onset
Functional decline

Figure 4.1 The early course of schizophrenia is characterized by sequential premorbid, and prodromal phases before the psychotic episode sets in. This is followed frequently by recurrent relapses and remissions (transitional phase) followed by a chronic, stable phase

is variable, with many patients showing persistent negative symptoms and cognitive deficits, and/or recurrent psychotic or affective episodes.

Psychotic disorders are common, with a lifetime prevalence of 3–4%. The prevalence of schizophrenia is slightly under 1% (McGrath, 2004; Saha et al., 2005); thus, about 3 million people in the United States have schizophrenia. Other psychotic disorders include substance-induced psychotic conditions, depression and bipolar disorder with psychotic features, and psychoses due to medical causes (such as head injury and temporal lobe epilepsy). Schizophrenia is often highly disabling and life-altering for patients and their families. Due to its typical emergence during later adolescence or early adulthood, schizophrenia can interrupt crucial milestones of young adult development, rob people of their autonomy and productivity during their prime working years, and can interfere with their capacity to form meaningful relationships.

According to the World Health Organization, schizophrenia ranks as one of the top ten global causes of years lost to disability, for both men and women. Schizophrenia occurs in both sexes, though males have a slightly higher (about a 1.4-factor elevated) risk of schizophrenia compared to females. The disorder can occur throughout the lifespan, but the period of greatest risk occurs in later adolescence and early adulthood. Prevalence rates are somewhat lower in developing countries. Outcomes for schizophrenia may be better in developing countries compared to developed countries. A mix of biological and environmental factors impart risk for developing the illness. Schizophrenia is more prevalent in urban than rural areas, a finding initially thought to result from a "drift" of people with the illness to urban areas. While some studies suggest that urban birth and upbringing are associated with an increased risk of schizophrenia because of factors such as higher urban levels of social stress, air pollution, vitamin D deficiency, prenatal infections, and cannabis use, urban–rural differences are generally modest in psychiatric disorders and still controversial. Prevalence of schizophrenia may be about three times higher in immigrants compared with native populations. While risk in European countries appears highest for Afro-Caribbean and other African immigrant groups, the countries of origin of these groups do not show increased prevalence rates. Experiences of social stress, discrimination, and poverty have been suggested as potential mechanisms, as well as delayed exposure to infectious pathogens not present in the country of origin. Further studies are needed to evaluate these theories more specifically.

Genetic factors are among the most well-known risk factors for psychotic disorders. A large number of genes are likely to be involved, which interact with several environmental factors to cause the vulnerability to these illnesses. Large-scale genome-wide association studies have revealed that a large number of these genes are involved in governing brain development, immune function, neurotransmitter systems such as glutamate (not just dopamine) and nerve cell conduction. Other risk factors include obstetrical complications, especially hypoxia which almost doubles the risk of schizophrenia, and increased paternal age perhaps due to an increased rate of mutations during spermatogenesis in older men. People born in the winter or early spring appear to have a slightly greater risk of schizophrenia compared to those born at other times of the year. Incidence of schizophrenia is higher in individuals born in the 4–5 months after influenza epidemics, suggesting that prenatal exposure to infections may be a risk factor.

4.2 Therapeutic Setting and Assessment

Patients who are referred for cognitive rehabilitation are often those that have been recently discharged from their first or a subsequent hospitalization, or have been referred by another treater, and are therefore likely to be in a transitional phase. Increasingly, patients referred to these programs are those in the early course of a psychotic disorder and are therefore new to the mental health system. In recent years, there is an increasing focus on developing coordinated specialty care programs that integrate multiple elements of treatment (such as psychopharmacology, supported employment, psychotherapy, peer engagement, and family-focused treatment). When implemented in a team setting, such programs are more likely to enhance therapeutic outcome and improve quality of life, as evidenced by the results of the Recovery After Initial Schizophrenia Episode (RAISE) study (Kane et al., 2015). The effectiveness of therapeutic approaches such as cognitive enhancement is likely to be amplified if embedded in such an integrated therapeutic context (Figure 4.2; Kline & Keshavan, 2017).

A comprehensive approach needs to be taken for the initial assessment. New requests for the same historical information that they have already shared with other clinicians are likely to frustrate patients. It is therefore important to get permissions for medical record releases from them such that as much as possible of the prior medical information can be obtained and reviewed close to the initial assessment. Careful attention to the following aspects of history should be obtained: prior episodes of psychotic illness, triggers for relapse and the individual's characteristic prodromal signs; prior treatments, responses, compliance, and side effects; comorbid medical or substance use, affective disorders; family and other support systems, prior psychosocial interventions (or lack thereof); and patient strengths.

There is often the tendency among clinicians not to obtain critically needed family input on key aspects of the patient's illness and prior care because of issues of the need to preserve confidentiality. Such misplaced altruism and overemphasis on HIPAA rules can actually impede comprehensive assessment (Hogarty, 2002). The time of first assessment offers an opportunity to set the tone for a collaborative relationship between family and significant others, treaters and the patient and create an open communication loop such

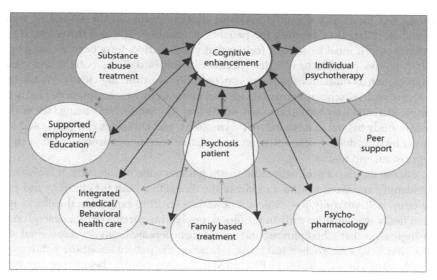

Figure 4.2 Cognitive enhancement interventions work best when embedded in a Coordinated Specialty Care Program

that all are part of the patient's treatment team. Patient concerns about confidentially can be addressed by giving examples of what type of information will be shared and why, and offering the patient the opportunity to set limits on sharing certain types of information (for instance, details about what occurs in each therapy session).Often, valuable information for treatment planning can be obtained with input from other team members, (e.g. patient's functional impairments at place of work may be best elicited during discussions with a supported employment therapist, and medication non-adherence may be evident to the case manager who interacts with group-home staff. Coordinated care team meetings are therefore very helpful in facilitating timely and valuable communications between team members (Figure 4.2).

4.3 Alliance and Engagement

Therapeutic alliance is critically important for successful outcomes in psychotherapy. Frank and Gunderson (Frank & Gunderson, 1990) examined the relationship between positive therapeutic alliance and favorable outcome in the early course of schizophrenia. In this important study, patients who had good alliance with their therapists within the first 6 months of treatment remained in psychotherapy more frequently, had better adherence to medications, and had better outcomes after 2 years.

Several key elements are to be considered in establishing a positive therapeutic alliance. First, many patients have limited insight into their illness and do not perceive the need for ongoing treatment. Xavier Amador (Amador, 2010) has articulated a very useful framework for helping clinicians develop a trusting therapeutic relationship, the LEAP principle. This involves active *listening*, accurate *empathy*, developing an *agreed* upon set of goals, and a *plan* based on shared decision-making. Early in the illness, patients may prefer to avoid prolonged discussions about the content of psychotic symptoms but the clinician should make an effort to point out the associated feelings. For example, rather than labeling the patients' paranoid beliefs and delusions, it would be better to say "it must be hurtful feeling that your relatives have been plotting against you," it is always possible to identify specific difficulties that the patient and clinician both agree, such as difficulties in sleep, concentration, or thinking clearly. We also avoid using terms such as schizophrenia (which has many negative connotations) early on in the illness. Patients may have their own words they are comfortable using (see examples in the case study below) to describe their symptoms, and clinicians can gently add to this repertoire by introducing descriptive terms to define specific syndromes such as psychosis, depression, and mania.

In order to develop a productive and trusting therapeutic relationship, it is also important to identify and work toward a model of the illness that both the clinician and patient can *agree* upon. Thankfully, few clinicians nowadays resort to explaining the illness as arising from faulty relationships early in the illness, or blaming parents or other caregivers. It is increasingly clear that schizophrenia and related disorders are brain developmental abnormalities, and have a neurochemical basis. Educating the patient about the nature of such abnormalities can be a challenge, as illustrated in the case example below (see case study).

Case Study 4.1

Lucy, a 22-year-old woman, had been brought to one of us (MSK) for gradual social withdrawal, talking to herself, and beliefs that she is the messiah destined to eliminate poverty from the world. She had dropped out of electrical engineering in her sophomore college year because of failing grades and disinterest in attending classes. She had refused medications, and had only grudgingly agreed to see a psychiatrist. In her first session, she denied all psychotic symptoms, but admitted to being unhappy about dropping out of college. When queried about her experience in college, she said she liked the topic of her studies, but could not pay attention in classes because of her mind being "cluttered" because of "chatter" inside her head. MSK then engaged her in a discussion on the topic she was studying in her classes: radio and transistors. When asked about how an electrical engineer would explain why a radio is unable to tune into the right station and get a lot of "static", she readily pointed out the increase in noise and decrease in the signal. MSK then suggested the possibility that if her brain were like a radio out of tune, could it explain her inability to concentrate, and the chatter (or "static") inside her head. She was willing to consider this possibility. This then led MSK to explain how dopamine might govern the tuning function in the brain, and if unbalanced, it could explain her symptoms; and how a medicine such as aripiprazole could correct that imbalance. She then agreed to consider a small dose trial for a while.

4.4 Psychoeducation

Learning about one's own illness is a large part of coming to grips with it. The goals of psychoeducation are to obtain an accurate perspective on schizophrenia or another psychotic disorder as a treatable "no-fault" brain disease, so that unnecessary guilt, hopelessness, and blame can be avoided, and a rationale provided for a treatment plan that focuses on realistic short- and long-term goals. Psychoeducation needs to be *tailored* to the patient's level of recovery and ability to process information. Cultural beliefs about the causes of mental illness should also be asked about and, when possible, incorporated into (or acknowledged alongside of) clinical explanations for symptoms. Early in the psychotic illness, lack of insight, denial, and impaired attention may limit the ability to process information; formal psychoeducation sessions need to be scheduled therefore following stabilization of crises and acute symptoms. Interactive workshop-like formats can be economic and helpful. Education needs to be offered in an *optimistic* tone, highlighting the therapeutic options available. Explaining what we know of the pathophysiology of the illnesses, and how treatments address such pathophysiology can be very helpful (e.g. dopamine imbalance and how antipsychotics correct such imbalance); using diagrams and other visual aids to explain such principles can be very effective. Given the cognitive limitations of attention and memory, it is important to *reintroduce* psychoeducation periodically during follow up, and whenever opportunities arise. An effective way to ensure comprehension of the learnt material is to elicit feedback about key concepts at the end of each session. Teaching about the illness also needs to be *gradual*, with the more neutral topics discussed first (e.g. sleep, nutrition) and contentious topics such as delusions and medication compliance at a later date as the patient is beginning to develop more trust.

4.5 Material and Psychological Support

Several studies point to the efficacy of supportive psychotherapy in schizophrenia though the precise definition of supportive psychotherapy has not been consistently provided. Supportive therapy includes correct empathy, appropriate reassurance, and opportunity for ventilation for the patient's distress in a non-judgmental setting. Interpretation is best avoided, and can often be perceived as criticism, which can be stressful. Supportive psychotherapy is often thought to represent "friendliness with a purpose"; however, the tendency to allow pathological transference and excessive dependence on therapists should be carefully avoided.

Material support is important in the early phases of stabilization, and this might involve help with case management, supportive housing, and assistance with income sources during the vulnerable period, such as Social Security Income (SSI) and Social Security Disability Income (SSDI). Clinicians are often faced with a dilemma as to whether too long a dependence on SSI/SSDI might engender dependence and slow recovery, but a careful assessment by the clinician about the phase of recovery and the nature of available support systems will enable the best decisions to be made collaboratively with the patient and care providers.

4.6 Coping with and Reducing Stress

As Joseph Zubin (Zubin, 1977) elegantly posited many decades ago, schizophrenia and other psychotic disorders are best conceptualized as illnesses that result from an inherent vulnerability that interacts with stress. In this model, individuals vary on a continuum between those with low vulnerability who only develop symptoms when faced with overwhelming stress, and those with high vulnerability who have breakdowns with even minimal stress (Figure 4.3). A useful way to explain this concept to patients and family members is by using the *Bucket* model; in this model, a smaller bucket (high vulnerability) will fill up even with little rain and begin to overflow, while a larger bucket (low vulnerability) can tolerate larger amounts of rain before it begins to overflow (Figure 4.4).

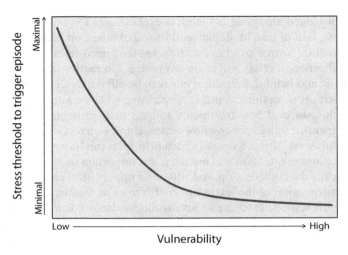

Figure 4.3 The stress vulnerability model by Joseph Zubin (see Zubin and Spring, 1977)

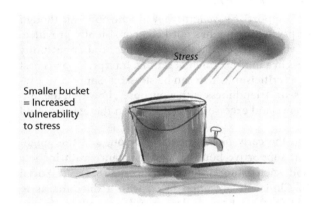

Figure 4.4 The bucket model for educating patients about stress and vulnerability

Psychoeducation needs to focus both on getting patients learn their own unique signs of relapse, and to monitor their own typical triggers of what makes symptoms to recur. Giving them an early warning symptoms and signs checklist is useful (see Table 4.2).

Early in the course of stabilization of psychotic disorders, the patients are more likely to be internally preoccupied, and because of the poor insight and denial, the clinician's approach to stress management has to be more general, i.e. reassurance, enlisting family support, therapist availability, and medications as needed. As acute symptoms subside, however, simple strategies such as teaching the patients breathing exercises, distraction (e.g. music, walking), and guided imagery can be introduced. It would be useful to encourage patients to identify individually unique imagery that might be effective in reducing stress. A patient treated by one of us (MSK) had figured that visualizing a calm ocean landscape was the best way to ward off his visual hallucinations; he always kept

Table 4.2 Early warning symptoms and signs of relapse (Birchwood, Spencer, & McGovern, 2000; Hogarty, 2002)

Affect	Behavior	Cognition/thinking
Feeling anxious and restless	Disorganized speech	Thoughts are racing
Feeling irritable	Talking or smiling to yourself	Thinking you have special powers
Feeling sad or low	Neglecting your appearance	Thinking others can read your mind or
Feeling confused or puzzled	Not eating	you can read others' minds
Feeling overwhelmed	Not socializing	Thinking others are against you. Thinking
Feeling like you cannot trust	Behaving aggressively	people are talking about you
people	Not leaving the house	Having unusual thoughts
Feeling like being watched	Difficulty sleeping	Thoughts are racing
Feeling increasingly religious	Drinking more	Senses seem sharper
Feeling tired or having low	Smoking more	Seeing visions others don't see
energy	Movements are slow	Hearing sounds others don't hear
		Feeling your body has changed
		Difficulty concentrating
		Trouble making decisions

a postcard with a beautiful seascape in his shirt pocket. It is also helpful to introduce consistent routines (habits) which create a safe environment; knowing in advance the expected daily tasks. This makes these tasks automatic and less effortful, and therefore less stressful. While having daily routines is useful for everyone, it is particularly helpful for patients who have trouble remembering specific tasks, or have difficulty in figuring what the next steps are in a given situation.

Stress elicits an activation of the sympathetic nervous system, thereby triggering a wide range of bodily responses such as increasing heart rate and muscle tension. By contrast, activation of the parasympathetic system leads to a reduction of such responses. There is a large body of evidence that use of relaxation and deep breathing techniques, which developed in eastern spiritual traditions, can be particularly helpful in reducing the stress response in a variety of psychiatric disorders. There are several techniques that involve voluntarily regulated breathing practices (VRBPs). Slow VRBPs tend to be relaxing and rapid, forceful VRBPs tend to increase alertness (Brown, Gerbarg, & Muench, 2013). We use a deep breathing approach that involves about 4 seconds inhalation through both nostrils, holding breath for 2 seconds, exhalation for 6 seconds, and 2 seconds of a pause before the next breathing cycle. This 4-2-6-2 cycle, which is about four cycles per minute, induces calm, and activates the parasympathetic system. The patient is asked to keep his hand over his belly while engaging in this breathing practice, to ensure diaphragmatic breathing (Kabat-Zinn, 1996). Patients are taught this approach during their therapeutic sessions, and then asked to routinely perform this practice while resting at home sitting or lying down one or two times each day, 5–10 minutes at a time; with practice, they are able to use this technique while standing or walking, and in stressful situations. They can also be taught to use a repetitive, personally meaningful word or phrase (a mantra), or use a calming visual image while engaging in this practice in order to refocus the mind away from distressing thoughts.

A particular source of stress for patients with serious mental illnesses is being exposed to high levels of expressed emotion in their family members or significant others, notably criticism. This increases autonomic arousal, can worsen symptoms, and may lead to relapse. An important focus of treatment is to teach patients about criticism management skills. This includes coaching in mindful listening to the critic's comments and tone of voice, understanding the perspective of the critic (whether the criticism is valid or not), and generating an appropriate response. For details, the reader is encouraged to read Gerard Hogarty's volume on PT (Hogarty, 2002).

4.7 Managing Comorbid Depression, Medical Illness, and Alcohol and Drug Abuse

Depressive symptoms are common, and often emerge or are "revealed" as the psychotic symptoms stabilize. These symptoms should be distinguished from negative symptoms, or medication side effects such as drug-induced Parkinsonism. Early identification and management of comorbid depression with pharmacological treatment (see Chapter 7) and psychotherapeutic approaches are critical.

Drug and alcohol abuse are significant problems for the population at large, but they pose special challenges for schizophrenia patients, as substance abuse decreases the likelihood that patients will follow recommended treatment plans, consequently leading to relapses. Patients may use drugs and alcohol to "self-medicate," to "escape" from the frustrating reality of chronic illness, or to create a social network with other users. Regardless of reasons for use, it can have many damaging effects. Incorporating motivational interviewing and harm reduction goals into routine psychotherapy for schizophrenia is important. Referring outpatients for separate substance use counseling can create problems with poorly coordinated care and even conflicting or inappropriate guidance on sobriety (for instance, some substance use programs discourage the use of prescribed psychiatric medications). Patients who enter treatment without a substance use problem should receive psychoeducation about how substances may exacerbate illness and threaten recovery goals.

4.8 Dealing with Dysfunctional Thoughts

Many people with serious mental illnesses have common distortions in thinking patterns which can be quite debilitating. Such maladaptive thinking is common in the early course of psychosis and may also emerge during cognitive enhancement treatments and can interfere with progress in therapy. In such patients, principles of Cognitive Behavior Therapy (CBT) are particularly helpful. Table 4.3 outlines common patterns of

Table 4.3 Self-defeating thoughts

Thought	Type of cognitive distortion
If I can't do this exercise, how can I ever get back to school?	Catastrophizing
I am a loser.	Labeling
I am a complete failure because I failed this test.	Black and white thinking
You should always try to be perfect.	Shoulds
When people are talking quietly, they are talking about me.	Personalization bias
Though my supervisor said I am a good employee, all I can remember is that one time when I made a mistake at work.	Filtering
A lot of people here are smarter than me.	Mind-reading

dysfunctional thoughts and examples. Several decades ago Aaron T. Beck developed CBT as a psychotherapeutic approach to address such self-defeating beliefs in major depressive disorder. There is evidence that CBT is effective for positive and negative symptoms of schizophrenia (Rector & Beck, 2012). Details of this approach are beyond the scope of this chapter. Briefly, in CBT, patients and clinicians collaboratively identify the connections between automatic thoughts, mood, and behavior. The therapist then helps the patient to reframe such thoughts in a neutral or positive light.

4.9 Resuming Daily Tasks and Improving Functionality

Patients with schizophrenia frequently find it hard to maintain focus over longer periods of time, indicating a lack of mental stamina, especially early in the illness. For this reason, it is best to resume functioning gradually. We often operate under the principle of *one change at a time*, and early during stabilization of the illness, the focus has to be on reinstituting self-care, including nutrition and personal hygiene. Gradually simple household responsibilities can be resumed, initially with collaboration by other family members, and later independently. Large projects should be broken down into smaller tasks, tackling each small piece one at a time, completing the one smaller task before moving on to the next one (e.g. not trying to clean the whole apartment all at one time). The patient may gradually resume earlier educational or vocational goals, but here again in a step-wise manner. Discussions with college counselors and employers for making accommodations at school/work can be helpful. Letting patients know to expect setbacks (*two steps forward and one step back*), and also to avoid unnecessary comparisons with others would be valuable. Patients often tend to blame themselves for not getting ahead and compare themselves unfavorably with their peers who did not develop the illness. A useful strategy, used in PT and in CET (Chapter 6), is to teach patients to avoid comparing themselves to others, but to evaluate and acknowledge their own progress relative to early periods of their illness when they were much more ill (*the internal yardstick concept*).

Many schizophrenia symptoms make it challenging for patients to communicate effectively with others at home, school, or work. Paranoid or suspicious thoughts may cause them to be fearful of others, while medications may make them too sleepy to sustain conversation. Even interactions that do occur may be disrupted by the inability to process information or the ability to carry through on plans due to apathy. Social skills training that can help address this challenge, should be part of the overall treatment plan.

4.10 Integration and Adjustment to Disability

There are multiple phases of recovery in people with serious mental illnesses, as illustrated in Figure 4.5 (Tse et al., 2014). Alan's case (see case study below) illustrates the phases of recovery. First is *symptomatic recovery* which Alan appears to have accomplished, and the second is *functional recovery*, in which he has made some progress with his improvements in cognitive function and motivation. However, the third phase is *personal recovery* which Alan is still struggling with, and refers to a person's ability to live a meaningful life despite the limitations of mental illness. These phases of recovery are related to each other and complementary, but require the therapist to be aware that true recovery may take years, even after symptomatic and functional remission.

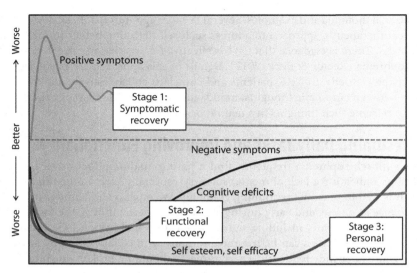

Figure 4.5 Stages of recovery in schizophrenia and related disorders

---

Case Study 4.2

Alan is a 26-year-old single Filipino man with schizoaffective disorder. He has recovered well from his symptoms after two hospitalizations that began when he was in college at age 22. His symptoms included delusions that he was being wiretapped wherever he went, hallucinations of computer-like voices and inability to concentrate, leading him to drop out of a graphic arts school. Following two hospitalizations, his symptoms have now largely subsided with the exception of occasional anxiety in social situations and fleeting paranoid thoughts. His ability to concentrate in day-to-day activities has improved and he is now able to work in a coffee shop. He is also more motivated now, his mood is better, and he is able to socialize.

However, Alan feels his life has "really not moved forward." He is reluctant to go out on dates because of worries that he will have to deal with questions (such as what to say and what not to say) about his illness. While he realizes that risperidone has been helpful, he is considering stopping it because he feels that only people with no willpower use medicines to solve their problems. Additionally, Alan's family is critical of him not looking for jobs (even though he is an excellent graphic artist), and wants him to get a job and support himself, because of tight finances. Alan has recently begun going out with old friends to watch Sports on Saturday nights. Even though he knows he should not, he has noticed that he is drinking and occasionally smoking pot as his friends do. He laments that because of his illness he will not "fit in" his friend group, and will never get a girlfriend and marry, because "he is schizophrenic."

Clearly Alan's situation is an example of incomplete recovery. The therapist's work is cut out in Alan's case (see Hogarty, 2002). In a series of sessions, the therapist, by using role play, modelling, and rehearsal, helped Alan to avoid comparing himself to others and measure himself by his own accomplishments (the internal yardstick concept), helped him develop internal coping skills to anticipate and avoid getting anxious when going on dates or job interviews. He also helped Alan to see himself as more than schizophrenia, and become aware of his strengths as well as limitations. He helped Alan to practice mindful listening of his family's perspectives, to acknowledge valid criticisms, and to respond appropriately. Alan also became more aware of his own unique indicators of relapse, his habitual responses to stress, and began to either use his own coping mechanisms (such as diaphragmatic breathing) or to walk away from conflict when he could not resolve the conflicts. Alan finally got some job interviews and was indeed asked about his medical history by an employer. The therapist coached him to use some appropriate self-disclosure and put "his best foot forward" when asked about his illness ("I have schizophrenia, but I am well now, and my doctor thinks I am ready to get back to work").

4.11 Summary

- Schizophrenia and related disorders are characterized by psychotic, affective, and cognitive symptoms; stabilizing psychotic and affective symptoms is critically important before addressing the core cognitive deficits.
- Managing the early phase of these disorders requires a careful assessment, building an optimum therapeutic alliance, individually tailored psychoeducation and ensuring adequate material and psychotherapeutic support.
- Schizophrenia is best understood using a stress-vulnerability model. Identification of cues of distress and early warning signs, and learning coping techniques are critical for preventing relapse.
- Functional impairments are best addressed by a step-wise resumption of activity, beginning with safety and self-care, and progressing gradually to return to vocational or school activities.

Computer-based Approaches to Cognitive Enhancement

5.1 Introduction

The vast potential of the human brain to adapt and repair itself, along with the eluci-dation of focused principles for cognitive training (see Chapters 2 and 3), have led to considerable interest and advancement in computer-based approaches to cognitive enhancement. The early 2010s saw the introduction of the first television advertisements for cognitive training software, and there now exist dozens of commercially available applications purporting to improve such cognitive domains as attention, memory, and problem-solving for people with psychiatric conditions (Torous et al., 2016). Despite the rapid emergence of computerized programs designed to improve the brain and cogni-tive functions, the earliest cognitive training protocols were paper-and-pencil based (e.g. Brenner, 2000; Wykes et al., 1999). These training programs were simple, but effective, and used worksheets, puzzles, and basic cognitive tasks (e.g. finger sequencing) without the aid of a computer. Further, research evidence in schizophrenia indicates that comput-erized programs are no more effective than old-fashioned paper-and-pencil approaches (Wykes et al., 2011). What computers do allow, however, is the easy standardization of training routines and automatic progression through exercises, which has facilitated the widespread use of these programs throughout psychiatry, the field of mental health, and indeed, the general public.

Although computerized approaches put cognitive training protocols in the hands of many more people than would have otherwise had access to such treatment, they do not eliminate the need for a mental health professional or a "coach" to support train-ing and help ensure that cognitive gains are translated to everyday life. Some computer-ized approaches are nearly fully self-administered, such as Posit Science (now known as brainHQ). They require some assistance from a technician or clinician to set up and enroll in the training program, but are largely self-directed from there on out. Other approaches, such as those employed in Cognitive Enhancement Therapy, rely on the use of an in-session coach to help guide participants through the training, to encourage strategic thinking, and to facilitate the generalization of cognitive gains to meaningful functional activities. Both approaches appear to be equally effective at improving basic cognitive processes in schizophrenia and related disorders (e.g. Fisher et al., 2009a; Hogarty et al., 2004). However, there is growing recognition by the field that some coaching or bridging by a mental health professional is likely to be necessary to support improved real-world functioning (Goldberg et al., 2010), The rationale being that simply improving a cognitive ability is not enough to ensure that the ability is used and used wisely. The appropriate use of cognitive skills based on situational demands is a metacognitive domain in which people with schizophrenia experience considerable difficulty (Lysaker et al., 2015; see Chapter 1), and coaching is often helpful for ensuring that individuals make the most out of their newfound cognitive skills.

The plethora of computerized training programs available can make it difficult for users and patients to decide which program might be best for them. Although professional game developers and other software companies have a rapidly growing supply of "brain training" programs, only a handful of suites have been evaluated and demonstrated benefit for improving cognition in schizophrenia. This chapter will provide an overview of these different training programs, their therapeutic targets, and their implementation with people with schizophrenia and related disorders. We describe below some of the computer cognitive training programs commonly used in schizophrenia.

5.2 Orientation Remedial Module (1982)

The Orientation Remedial Module (ORM) was developed in the 1980s by Yehuda Ben-Yishay at New York University for the amelioration of attentional problems in people suffering from head trauma and brain injury (Ben-Yishay, Piasetsky, & Rattok, 1985). The program was designed to help "shape" attention through the use and gradual fading of cues, both auditory and visual. The general approach of the ORM is to ask participants to engage in a series of exercises that require them to inhibit distraction and/or focus their attention for longer periods of time. Initially, cues are given to ease the difficulty of the exercise (e.g. the computer holds your attention for you), which are gradually removed based on certain performance criteria. The coach is careful to begin the exercise at a level of difficulty that is challenging, but achievable by the participant – a principle in cognitive training known as *scaffolding* (see Chapter 3). Once the participant gains some mastery, the difficulty of the exercise is increased by fading cues previously provided by the computer. Such cues now need to be internalized by the participant, requiring increased reliance on the self and use of attention.

Many computerized cognitive training programs utilize *scaffolding* to begin training and *cueing/fading* to adjust difficulty levels to match the cognitive abilities of the participant. An example of one of the ORM exercises, *Time Estimates*, helps to illustrate these principles. In this exercise of sustained attention, the participant is asked to view a clock with a single hour hand that sweeps around in a clockwise fashion when the space bar is pressed (see Figure 5.1).

When the space bar is released, the hour hand stops, and the goal of the exercise is to stop the hand precisely at 12:00. Two cues are available to help scaffold difficulty to the appropriate level of the participant. Auditory cues provide a simple beep when the hour hand passes an hour on the clock, and visual cues display the hour hand as it is sweeping around the clock. The hour hand sweeps across a 1-hour marker each second, and

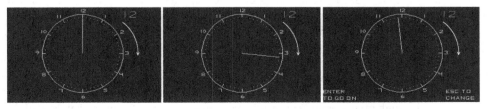

Figure 5.1 Time Estimates – example exercise from the Orientation Remedial Module (ORM)

typically cues are provided for the first 10 seconds, with the participant being required to hold their attention for the final 2 seconds to stop at 12:00. Initially, scaffolding is used to determine the level of cueing needed by the participant. Individuals with more cognitive challenges in attention may require both visual and auditory cues when beginning the exercise, whereas others may begin with only auditory cueing. This sets the initial difficulty level of the exercise to the capabilities of the participant so that training begins with success. Training programs that do not scaffold difficulty levels as a method of individualizing training to the participant's abilities are thought to have greater risk of negative outcomes, including disengagement, demoralization, and attrition. It is essential that cognitive training for individuals with schizophrenia begin at a difficulty level that is challenging, but one that the trainee can succeed at, to promote engagement and positive reinforcement for the training.

Cueing and fading is another essential principle in cognitive training that is illustrated by the *Time Estimates* exercise. Recall that in this exercise participants receive auditory or visual cues to help fixate their attention on the sweep of the hour hand. At the beginning of the exercise scaffolding sets the skill level to a relatively easy level of difficulty, where cues are provided for the first 10 seconds, and the participant must use their own "internal cueing" to maintain attention for the final 2 seconds at stop the hour hand at 12:00. As the exercise progresses, visual cues are faded almost immediately so that only auditory cues remain. Then, auditory cues are gradually faded two at a time until only four cues (beeps) are left (from 1:00 to 4:00), and participants learn to maintain their attention using their own internal resources for the remainder of the sweep (from 5:00 to 12:00), requiring significant sustaining of attention. Of course, this progression moves at a slow pace individualized to the participant, and usually requires four or more sessions in people with schizophrenia to achieve the highest difficulty level.

All of the exercises in the ORM are focused on training some aspect of processing speed or attention. Processing speed tasks are similar to those focused on attention, but require a fast, immediate response rather than careful sustaining of attention toward a particular stimulus. The ORM has been one of the most widely used computerized cognitive enhancement programs for people with schizophrenia, and studies have repeatedly shown it to be effective for improving processing speed and attention domains in this population (Eack et al., 2015; Hogarty et al., 2004).

5.3 PSSCogRehab (1982/2012)

Psychological Software Services by Bracy and colleagues has been developing cognitive rehabilitation software for brain and cognitive disorders for many years, and the PSSCogRehab suite is another set of computerized cognitive remediation programs that were originally developed for patients with traumatic brain injury and stroke. Since its initial development, PSSCogRehab has been widely applied to these populations, as well as to learning disabilities, attention deficit disorder, and individuals living with schizophrenia. Unlike the ORM, PSSCogRehab focuses on attention, memory, and problem-solving training within a comprehensive suite of exercises. Memory and problem-solving training have been most commonly used with patients with schizophrenia, as in Cognitive Enhancement Therapy (Hogarty & Greenwald, 2006). Difficulty settings are not as customizable as the ORM, and there are not as many opportunities with PSSCogRehab to fade cues, although most exercises have adjustable initial settings to appropriately scaffold the task to the ability level of the participant. In many cases, the practice of cueing/fading is secondary to teaching strategic thinking, as PSSCogRehab is perhaps most effective at enhancing higher-order cognitive processes in memory and executive function.

For example, one exercise in the PSSCogRehab suite is *Objects and Locations*, a memory routine that is designed to strengthen spatial working memory and promote strategic encoding of information to facilitate later recall. In this exercise, the participant views a 5 × 6 grid array of unrelated objects (see Figure 5.2), and is asked to remember a variable number of objects (e.g. 4) for a customizable study period (e.g. 4 seconds per object). During the study period, only the objects to be remembered appear on the screen, after which all 30 objects are visible and the participant must recall which items were presented for her to remember. The exercise can be appropriately scaffolded by adjusting object number and study time parameters, but otherwise the systematic fading of cues is not possible or necessary for training. Rather, participants must begin to learn to think strategically about how to encode information, as a pure reliance on verbatim memory is not sufficient to succeed in the exercise with greater numbers of objects (e.g. 8 or more). As the number of objects to be remembered grows, the possibility of succeeding in the exercise simply by holding the object in working memory becomes less and less feasible. Not only does working memory need to be strengthened by repeated practice, but also the exercise needs to be approached *strategically* to succeed and participants are encouraged to think and test out strategies that might improve encoding and retrieval.

In many cases, relational encoding is the critical strategy for memory exercises such as *Objects and Locations*. This encoding strategy teaches participants about the relational nature of memory stores (Mayes, Montaldi, & Migo, 2007), and how information is more easily recalled when it is connected with other information to be remembered. For example, if the participant was asked to recall pictures of the trumpet, boat, wheelbarrow, and violin in Figure 5.2, most would choose to store these words as more or less fixed and isolated representations in verbatim working memory. Unfortunately, the storage capacity of verbatim working memory is greatly limited and information decays rapidly once stored. As such, the participant will find difficulty in accurately recalling these items as the number of items and study time increases. Relational encoding of information can be introduced as a strategy to expanding working memory storage and enhancing retention. One simple way to use relational encoding during this exercise would be to construct a brief story about the items to be remembered. For example, Sam brought his *violin* on the *boat*, but forgot his *trumpet*, so he had to go back and pick it up with the *wheelbarrow*. In constructing such a story, these four words are no longer isolated, but are encoded relationally as pieces to a rather unusual and memorable narrative. Consequently, the information now requires some more effort to store (e.g. development of a gistful story), but is far easier to recall and allows for many more items to be remembered.

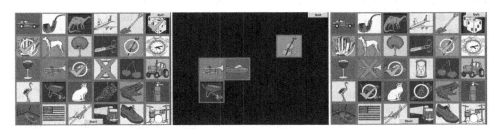

Figure 5.2 Objects and Locations – example exercise from PSSCogRehab

The focus of PSSCogRehab on higher-order cognitive exercises in memory and problem-solving makes it an excellent suite for facilitating strategic training. Participants not only have the opportunity to exercise working memory and other executive functions, but they also are confronted with tasks whose optimal solutions require planning, strategy, and critical thinking. In schizophrenia, these skills are as important, if not more important than the specific cognitive domain being trained, and as participants move through the exercises, it is critical to promote a strategic approach to solving problems on the computer and in everyday life (see Chapter 3 for discussion of strategic training). Although the PSSCogRehab suite was developed in the early 1980s, it was recently updated in 2012 to modernize the platform, ensure its compatibility with newer systems, and update the graphical content. Some newer exercises have been introduced, but many remain the same with modern day enhancements, and Psychological Software Services continues to actively develop the suite.

The PSSCogRehab suite has been utilized in a large number of clinical trials of cognitive remediation programs for people with schizophrenia, including Cognitive Enhancement Therapy (Hogarty et al., 2004). Previous studies have found significant improvements in attention, memory, and executive functioning associated with the use of the PSSCogRehab software when employed in a variety of cognitive enhancement programs (e.g. Bell et al., 2001; Bowie et al., 2012; Eack et al., 2009; Keefe et al., 2010).

5.4 Cogpack (1986)

Cogpack is perhaps the most widely used computerized cognitive remediation software for patients with schizophrenia. It has been a staple of intervention programs that have focused either on cognitive training alone or integrated it with broader psychosocial interventions (McGurk et al., 2007; Mueller, Schmidt, & Roder, 2015), and has considerable evidence for improving cognitive flexibility, verbal memory, and speed of processing in individuals with schizophrenia (e.g. Lindenmayer et al., 2008; McGurk et al., 2015). Like PSSCogRehab, Cogpack contains a broad suite of cognitive training exercises ranging from those designed to enhance vigilance and language, to routines focused on improving memory and problem-solving. Training proceeds in very much the same fashion as the ORM and PSSCogRehab, with scaffolding initial difficulty levels to the participant's ability, and then cueing/fading to increase difficulty with an increasing focus on strategic thinking and problem-solving as training ensues.

Figure 5.3 illustrates an example of vigilance and memory exercise implemented in Cogpack known as *Eye Witness*. This training routine is focused on improving vigilance, speed of processing, and visual memory and presents the participant with an animated scene of buildings, cars, names, and other objects. The participant studies the scene and the interactions among its contents for a brief period, and then is asked a series of questions about what took place (e.g. "How many vehicles passed?"). The participant is allotted as much time as necessary to answer the questions, but only has a limited time to study the contents of the scene being presented. In this way, she has to remain attentive and vigilant during the scene to be an accurate eye witness to its events. Customization of task difficulty can be accomplished by selecting the "easier" or "harder" settings, which controls the speed at which the scene is presented. This exercise is an example of the training of integrated cognitive abilities in vigilance, processing speed, and working memory, which affords many opportunities for strategic thinking around optimizing performance. Participants must clear their minds and focus on the fast-moving scene

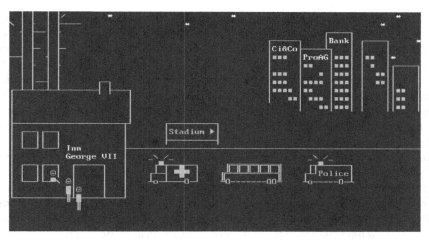

Figure 5.3 Eye Witness – example exercise from Cogpack

free from distraction, and then strategize how best to remember the information being presented. Relational encoding of information is often used as a strategy in this exercise (similar to *Objects and Locations* in PSSCogRehab) but is somewhat easier here, as the scene provides much of the context for developing a story around the information to be encoded (e.g. three people were staying at the George VII Inn before three vehicles came and picked them up). As participants complete the exercise successfully, they can also become more aware of the salient information they have to remember, and develop strategies to inhibit other distracting elements and focus on the key components of the scene.

In total, Cogpack contains 64 training routines across processing speed, attention/vigilance, memory, and problem-solving domains to provide a comprehensive neurocognitive training experience. The software also includes training routines in other domains that are not often included in neurocognitive programs, such as money management and how to read traffic signs. Although Cogpack was introduced in 1986, it has been continually developed to maintain interoperability with modern computing systems. Many of the exercises may appear dated by today's graphical standards, but they remain some of the most effective and widely used for enhancing basic neurocognitive abilities in patients with schizophrenia.

Cogpack has been one of the most widely studied (and utilized) computerized cognitive training programs in patients with schizophrenia. It has shown efficacy for improving many neurocognitive domains (Breitborde et al., 2015; Lindenmayer et al., 2008; Sartory et al., 2005), has been combined with supported employment programs to enhance their efficacy (e.g. McGurk et al., 2015), and combined with other individual and group-based approaches (e.g. Bowie et al., 2012). It remains a staple of computerized cognitive approaches to cognitive enhancement and has one of the largest evidence bases in the field.

5.5 Posit Science (2004)

Posit Science is the most modern of the neurocognitive training suites tested and shown to be effective for individuals with schizophrenia and related disorders. Originally developed by Merzenich and colleagues for dyslexia (Merzenich et al., 1996), Posit Science takes a very different approach to neurocognitive training than other available programs, by focusing on low-level auditory processing and its contribution to cognitive impairment in schizophrenia. Many years of basic neuroscience research conducted by Merzenich and colleagues demonstrated that early impaired auditory processing generates a noisy signal for the brain to interpret, leading to upstream deficits in higher-order cognitive abilities (e.g. Nagarajan et al., 1999). Patients with schizophrenia demonstrate such early sensory impairments (Javitt, Shelley, & Ritter, 2000), which are related to broader cognitive challenges (Javitt, 2009). The targeting of early sensory processing represents a true "bottom-up" approach.

Top-down approaches often focus on the remediation of higher-order systems first (e.g. working memory, problem-solving), with the expectation that lower-order processes will be improved as a result. Conversely, bottom-up approaches, such as the one employed by Posit Science, predict that by remediating early deficits in sensory inputs, higher-order system can then receive a cleaner neural signal, resulting in fewer cognitive challenges. In practice, both approaches appear to be helpful in addressing cognitive impairments in schizophrenia (Wykes et al., 2011), and Posit Science offers a significant advance in remediation protocols by providing sensory training in auditory processing as a bottom-up approach to treatment. Numerous studies have found this approach to be effective for enhancing cognition in schizophrenia, particularly in the domains of verbal learning and memory (Fisher et al., 2009a; Fisher, Achilles, & Tonnies, 2014).

The Posit Science Corporation develops several cognitive training routines and packages. Brain Fitness was their primary auditory training program that has now been included in the more comprehensive suite from the company, brainHQ, which provides attention, memory, and other neurocognitive exercises. Figure 5.4 gives a visual example of *Sound Sweeps*, one of the main auditory training programs in brainHQ. In this simple, yet challenging exercise, the participant is asked to wear a set of headphones in/through which a series of tones will be played. The tones will either start at a lower pitch and then increase or vice versa, and the participant is tasked with identifying whether the tone is playing "high or low." The sweeping of the tone across frequencies moves on a millisecond scale, making the task quite challenging and a real test for early auditory processing. Beyond the advance of the new early sensory training approach employed in brainHQ, Posit Science was also one of the first neurocognitive programs to implement automatic computerized adjustments to task difficulty based on assessment and performance. In the case of *Sound Sweeps*, the duration of the sweep and the interval between tones is automatically adjusted by the computer to maintain a high level of

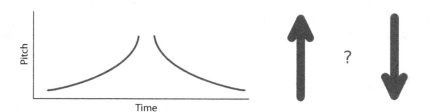

Figure 5.4 Sounds Sweep – example exercise from brainHQ by Posit Science

performance (~85% accuracy), which keeps participants engaged in the task, scaffolds difficulty to their ability level, and automates much of the training process.

Although brainHQ offers a variety of training exercises in several domains, the auditory training programs have been the most studied in patients with schizophrenia, indicating that enhancing early auditory processing is associated with significant improvements in global cognition, and verbal learning and memory (Fisher et al., 2009a). Because of the automated and web-based nature of the program, it is becoming more feasible for individuals to complete neurocognitive training at home or away from the clinic using laptops and tablet computers, which has recently been shown to be effective for patients in the early course of schizophrenia (Fisher et al., 2015).

5.6 Lumosity (2007)

An emerging computer-based neurocognitive training suite that has received much popular attention is Lumosity. A spin-off from Posit Science, Lumosity aims to bring cognitive training to the masses and has been one of the most commonly advertised suites for "brain training" available. The suite contains numerous activities and exercises, ranging from basic lower-order processing and attentional abilities, to higher-order task shifting and problem-solving skills. The suite is highly customizable, based on a personalized baseline assessment, and has been developed with high-quality human interface design and artwork, making Lumosity one of the most user-friendly and engaging cognitive training programs. The efficacy of the suite for schizophrenia and other neuropsychiatric conditions remains to be established, however initial studies have shown promise (Hooker et al., 2014).

5.7 CIRCuiTS

Another promising approach to computer-based neurocognitive training is Computerized Interactive Remediation of Cognition – a Training for Schizophrenia (CIRCuiTS), which focuses on strategy-based training in attention, memory, and executive functioning. Particularly unique to CIRCuiTS is the embedding of different cognitive exercises within ecologically valid tasks, such as cooking and shopping, in an effort to bridge cognitive and functional gains. CIRCuiTS is strategy-based in which participants are actively encouraged to develop strategies to improve and regulate their cognitive abilities, and the program also emphasizes the development of metacognitive abilities through assessment and discussion with a clinician. Initial evidence has suggested that this emerging computer-based approach is effective at improving memory and executive functioning in patients with schizophrenia, with increases in time spent in structured activities also observed associated with treatment with CIRCuiTS (Reeder et al., 2017). The approach represents one of the first attempts in computer-based training to develop more ecologically valid tasks for training cognition that can further assist in generalizing gains to functional outcomes.

5.8 Computer-based Social Cognition Training

To date, computer-based approaches to cognitive training for patients with schizophrenia have focused largely on the neurocognitive domains of attention, memory, and problem-solving. Posit Science is a notable exception for also developing training exercises in early sensory processing. That these cognitive processes are basic and non-social makes computerized approaches feasible for implementing repeated exercises designed to enhance these abilities, but what about cognitive deficits that are more social in nature? As reviewed in Chapter 1, patients with schizophrenia experience a broad range of cognitive impairments, including those in social cognition, or the ability to process and interpret socio-emotional information in oneself and others. Because these challenges emerge in social situations, the feasibility of utilizing computer-based approaches to improve social information processing may be limited. On the other hand, the wide availability of affordable computing and access to training software makes computerized approaches attractive for enhancing access to social cognition training programs.

Some notable computer-based approaches to training various social-cognitive processes have begun to emerge in scientific literature. Most of these programs focus on a single area of social cognition, many of which target the recognition of emotion in human faces. Figure 5.5 provides an illustrative example from Paul Ekman's Micro Expressions Training Tools (Ekman, 2004). In this program, participants are provided with psychoeducation via instructional videos on how different facial elements change with the expression of basic emotions (e.g. sadness, fear, anger). After learning about "micro" changes in facial expressions, individuals are then asked to watch a brief scene where a person's facial expressions change from a neutral to an emotional expression on a millisecond timescale. The participant then selects from a list of basic emotions what specific emotion she believes was expressed in the scene. Correct responses receive additional psychoeducation on why the selection was accurate. The premise behind such training programs, of which there are now many that focus on facial expressions, is that learning the subtleties of this important social cue will significantly enhance social cognition and perhaps even remediate some of the social disability experienced by people with schizophrenia.

Several studies have reported use of the Micro Expressions Training Tools among individuals with schizophrenia for improving social cognition, and have found increases in accurately identifying emotions in faces (Russell, Chu, & Phillips, 2006) and managing emotions (Sacks et al., 2013), but no improvements in other areas of social cognition or functional outcome. Similar patterns are observed showing significantly improved recognition of emotions in faces after other computerized facial emotion perception training programs (Silver et al., 2004), indicating that this is a domain that can be significantly enhanced using computerized methods, although functional improvements have not often been evaluated or observed (Bordon, O'Rourke, & Hutton, 2017). Another emerging computer-based social cognition training program is SocialVille, developed by the Posit Science team. Socialville is a fully computerized social cognition training suite that aims to improve the speed and accuracy with which social information is processed. Exercises include emotion perception labeling, face matching, gaze identification and matching, and other aspects of emotion processing. To date, evidence suggests that SocialVille is feasible in young adults with schizophrenia, however efficacy has yet to be established in controlled trials (Nahum, Fisher, & Loewy, 2014). Computerized approaches to training social cognition clearly show challenges and opportunities as developers work to expand areas of training, improve generalization to social behavior, and identify novel ways to embed meaningful components of the social environment in training exercises. This is an emerging area of the

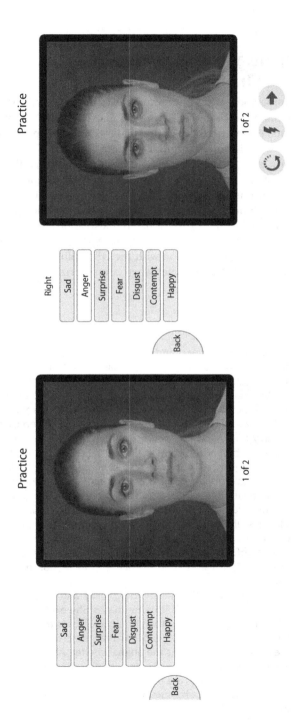

Figure 5.5 Micro Expressions Training Tools – computerized social cognition training example

field that is growing significantly and is likely to be increasingly integrated with individual and group-based approaches to cognitive training.

5.9 Optimizing Therapeutic Opportunities in Computer-based Training

Computer-based training approaches offer unparalleled access to exercises that are beneficial for addressing the neurocognitive, sensory, and even possibly some of the social-cognitive impairments experienced by individuals with schizophrenia. Approaches range from clinic-based, clinician/coach-guided training programs, such as in Cognitive Enhancement Therapy, to essentially fully automated programs that can be self-administered and do not rely on a mental health professional, such as brainHQ by Posit Science. Automated programs offer unique benefits in adaptive training, scalability, and anytime access. Clinician-guided training programs are more challenging to implement and require a trained mental health professional, but also afford therapeutic opportunities for enhancing strategic training and promoting generalization of learned skills. Larry and Aarav's neurocognitive training session with the ORM illustrates some ways a clinician can help optimize therapeutic outcomes when computerized training is guided by a professional.

Case Study 5.1

Larry has had schizophrenia for 20 years and is interested in improving his attention so that he can start volunteering at the animal shelter. Aarav is a young college senior with schizophrenia who is struggling to finish his degree in engineering. They are participating in Cognitive Enhancement Therapy, where one of the principles is to conduct neurocognitive training in participant pairs to facilitate motivation, engagement, and early socialization. Although their ages are different, the clinician has given careful thought into the pairing of Larry and Aarav for neurocognitive training. Neuropsychological testing revealed both have higher IQ scores (110–120s), but profound impairments in speed of processing and vigilance. They both also have a love for baseball, and Larry had previously attended college when he was younger. Aarav presents with significant impairments in motivation, whereas Larry has more of a disorganized cognitive style. Intellectual ability, areas of cognitive impairment, interests, and background experiences are all factors clinicians should use when pairing participants for training. Ultimately the clinician should decide what individuals are likely to make a successful pair, and it is also often helpful to avoid pairing two individuals with the same cognitive style (e.g. disorganized), as this can increase challenges in session management and progress during training.

The session begins with the clinician reminding Larry and Aarav of the cognitive exercise they are working on in the ORM, Time Estimates. She explains that this routine is designed to help them stay vigilant and then briefly discusses the role of vigilance in their respective goals. For Larry, the coach explains that exercise will help him stay on task and keep an eye on those puppies at the animal shelter. Aarav comments that he also sees how staying vigilant during class will help with his note-taking and understanding the class lectures. These discussions are essential for making a link between the basic cognitive abilities being trained, the behavioral skills they will ultimately support, and the individual's personal goals.

Larry is feeling up to the task and volunteers to start Time Estimates for the session. Aarav takes Larry's scoresheet and sits next him at the computer, so that he can help his partner keep score while he is working on the exercise. The clinician instructs Larry to begin, and as the exercise ensues Larry struggles to keep his focus on the sweeping hand of the clock (see Figure 5.1). Aarav offers some support, saying "Don't worry Larry, you got this!" Despite the words of encouragement, Larry is just feeling too excited and cannot keep focused. The clinician intercedes, commenting on Larry's struggles and giving positive reinforcement for his effort. "Larry, you are putting in a good effort. I noticed you are struggling some, though. Can you think of any strategies to help you stay focused?" Larry thinks back to a previous session he had with similar struggles, and remembers that stopping and taking a deep breath before starting the exercise seemed to help in the past, "Yes, maybe I should take a deep breath like before?" The clinician asks Socratically, "Why do you think that would be helpful?" Larry answers, "My mind isn't getting into it, it might help me focus." The clinician asks Larry to sit straight on his chair, close his eyes, put his hand over his diaphragm, and push out a couple of slow, deep breaths.

Larry returns to the exercise after taking a couple of relaxing deep breaths, and his first couple of trials are successful! The clinician provides reinforcement indicating that taking a deep breath appears to have been helpful in orienting his attention. Larry continues and struggles a bit more, with the coach, and occasionally Aarav, giving reminders to slow down, take a couple of deep breaths, and relax. His performance continues to improve and he successfully passes a level of Time Estimates.

This case example illustrates how optimal computer-based training can include much more than the participant sitting in front of a computer and repeatedly practicing the same exercise. Having a partner changes the training from an isolated task to a social one, with opportunities for empowerment, giving support, and enhancing motivation. In addition, as this example demonstrates, Larry and Aarav are learning much more than how to stop the sweep hand moving around a clock on Time Estimates. They are learning about attention and vigilance, and that they are working on these domains not just because a neuropsychological test indicated a deficit, but because they see how these deficits produce challenges in the real world and they want to overcome these challenges to achieve their goals of volunteering and finishing college. Further, Larry and Aarav are also learning the role of stress in cognition, a major factor in schizophrenia generally (Zubin & Spring, 1977), and how coping strategies such as deep breathing can make an immediate impact on performance. This moves neurocognitive training beyond a mere drill-and-practice approach to one that promotes strategic thinking and awareness of the factors that influence cognition. Such factors are then discussed in individual and group sessions, which are ideally integrated with computerized cognitive training to promote synergy among these components and enhance the generalization of treatment (see Figure 5.2). Consequently, there are many therapeutic opportunities in neurocognitive training, when led by a mental health professional, and practitioners should be vigilant to take advantage of such opportunities to maximize the translation of gains in computerized environments to broader aspects of daily life.

5.10 How to Select a Computer-based Neurocognitive Training Program

In recent years a large market has developed to meet the increasing demands of computer-based exercises in the field of cognitive remediation. An increasing range of programs are now available including local software based on hard drives, web-based programs available on computers, and as applications (or apps) on smart phones and tablets. Each of these programs has unique strengths and weaknesses based on the particular clinical needs; often individuals may need more than one program complementing each other. Clinicians therefore have to frequently make decisions for their patients and their clinical settings as to which among the various programs is most suitable. Such choices are best made by reviewing the prior evidence base showing the benefit of the program in the target population and keeping in mind the theoretical and practical framework of factors that underlie success with cognitive enhancement programs as discussed in Chapter 3. Briefly, these include the cost, usability, scalability, range of available exercises, motivational factors, and generalizability to living situations. Box 5.1 outlines a suggested approach to evaluate computer-based cognitive enhancement programs.

Box 5.1 Features to be assessed to determine suitability of a computer-based cognitive training program in clinical settings

Program features

1. Does the program have an established evidence base in the target population?
2. Does the program offer exercises that address cognitive domains in which the patient needs improvement?
3. Is the program scalable to unique patient features? (e.g. age, intellectual function, language)
4. Are the exercises contextualized to real life situations?
5. Are exercises offered that address a variety of contexts?
6. Do the exercises start with basic cognitive functions (e.g. sound discrimination), and proceed to more complex cognitive functions?
7. Are tips (e.g. strategic advice such as chunking) offered to enhance performance?
8. Are the exercises fun and interesting?
9. Does the program provide immediate feedback for task performance?
10. Are summary evaluations provided, and overall progress tracked over time?
11. Are rewards and points provided based on performance?
12. Do participants have choice in deciding type and difficulty level of exercise?
13. Do exercises automatically adjust to performance level?
14. Do exercises provide appropriate feedback for positive performance (congratulatory statements) and negative performance (support and reassurance)?
15. Is the program regularly updated based on user feedback?
16. Does the program allow for therapist involvement?
17. Is the program reasonably priced?
18. Is the program available in multiple platforms (e.g. CD, web-based, tablet, smartphone)

5.11 Summary

- Computer-based approaches for training neurocognitive domains of attention, memory, and problem-solving are effective in schizophrenia.
- Many different programs exist, but only a few have been scientifically evaluated: these include the ORM, PSSCogRehab, Cogpack, and Posit Science.
- Computerized methods of social cognition training are emerging, particularly training in the recognition of facial expressions of emotion, although more evidence is needed on generalization.
- Optimal neurocognitive training utilizes therapeutic opportunities in session to promote motivation, psychoeducation, and generalization of learned skills.
- In choosing a computer training program for a given patient, the clinician should consider several factors that underlie success with cognitive enhancement programs (see Box 5.1).

Individual and Group Approaches to Cognitive Enhancement

6.1 Introduction

The past decade has seen a surge in the development of computer-based approaches to cognitive training, and these programs offer standardized, portable, and easy-to-use methods for enhancing cognition in schizophrenia and related conditions. However, the earliest forms of cognitive training interventions used paper-and-pencil cognitive exercises without the aid of a computer (e.g. Brenner et al., 1994), and meta-analytic evidence indicates that basic paper-and-pencil approaches are equally as effective for improving cognition in schizophrenia as more advanced computerized methods (Wykes et al., 2011). As such, the computer should not be seen as the only or the critical therapeutic element in cognitive remediation, but rather an important tool for delivering and standardizing cognitive training protocols. While computer-based interventions are now common, it is important to recognize that many of the most effective cognitive training programs utilize individual and group-based approaches to improve social cognition, bridge skills learned during computer-based neurocognitive training, and integrate cognitive remediation into broader psychosocial treatment programs.

Individual and group approaches offer complementary methods for improving cognition and functional recovery to those employed in computer-based programs. Repeated practice of computerized routines to enhance attention, memory, and/or problem-solving is effective for enhancing many aspects of cognition in schizophrenia (e.g. Fisher et al., 2009a). Many clinicians recognize that patients engage well with the computer, enjoy a new treatment opportunity, and derive personal benefits from computerized training. However, it is also recognized that computer-based methods often leave little opportunity to discuss gained abilities, the transfer of skills learned on the computer to everyday settings, and the personalization of treatment to the pressing social and functional concerns of the patient. Even with the most effective and expertly automated computerized training program, there remains a clear need to speak with our patients about their goals, challenges, and progress in training (Fenton, 1997). Individual, one-on-one sessions are particularly helpful for addressing these issues.

Although it is well-known that most patients with schizophrenia experience cognitive challenges (Heinrichs & Zakzanis, 1998), there is a high degree of heterogeneity in the exact domains of impairment. Some individuals may have great difficulty with organization and working memory. Others may have challenges with mental stamina and a slow speed of processing. Hogarty and colleagues (Hogarty et al., 2004) introduced the concept of *cognitive styles* to recognize this heterogeneity and help the clinician personalize treatment to the particular style of the patient. Individual sessions with patients help to tailor treatment messages and computerized exercises to the areas of greatest impairment for a given person. For example, in CET, a person with an unmotivated cognitive style would often meet individually with their clinician to discuss the challenges that style presents to adaptive function and to direct computerized cognitive training toward the information processing impairments characterized by that style, such as a lack of motivation, reduced processing speed and mental stamina, and difficulty in planning. Individual sessions not only help tailor cognitive training to the specific abilities of the patient, but also help to provide the space and opportunity for discussions of how to use skills gained in cognitive remediation in everyday life to enhance functional outcomes such as employment, relationships, and school.

Group-based approaches are also a common component of cognitive training programs, especially those that seek to enhance social cognition. As discussed in Chapter 5, computer-based methods for enhancing social cognition are emerging, but concerns remain about the transfer of skills to real world social situations. However, a group setting is a powerful social situation that approximates the "real world" in many ways, including interacting with others in real time, learning from observing, responding to unrehearsed social exchanges, and managing anxiety associated with interacting with others in person. As such, many cognitive remediation approaches include a group-based component to improve social cognition, such as Cognitive Enhancement Therapy (CET; Hogarty & Greenwald, 2006), which has been shown to provide additional benefits to functioning when added to computer-based neurocognitive training (Hogarty et al., 2004; Mueller, Schmidt, & Roder, 2015). Programs that do not focus on social cognition also often employ group-based interventions to "bridge" skills learned during computerized training to everyday life, similar to individual approaches, but in a group format that can be more efficient and provide greater opportunity for socialization than an individual therapy session. This chapter will review the predominant individual and group-based approaches to cognitive remediation for schizophrenia and discuss their methods for enhancing social cognition and the transfer of learning from basic cognitive training exercises (see Table 6.1 for an overview of approaches).

6.2 Integrated Psychological Therapy (1980, 1994)

Integrated Psychological Therapy (IPT) is one of the first and most well-studied group-based cognitive remediation approaches for schizophrenia. Originally developed in Germany by Brenner and colleagues (Brenner et al., 1980, 1994), IPT is a comprehensive cognitive remediation intervention that integrates group-based neurocognitive training with group-based training in social cognition, social skills, and interpersonal problem-solving. Likely one of the most comprehensive cognitive remediation models to date, IPT seeks to address the neurocognitive and social-cognitive challenges in schizophrenia that underlie and maintain social dysfunction in the disorder. IPT takes a bottom-up hierarchical approach to address social functioning problems through five integrated treatment components or sub-programs (see Figure 6.1).

These treatment components first focus on targeting basic neurocognitive abilities, referred to as cognitive differentiation. Neurocognitive training in IPT is group-based and not computerized, and unlike many of the drill-and-practice computer-based approaches available today, IPT focuses less on repetition of a cognitive task and more on strategic planning and problem-solving. Basic cognitive exercises similar to those automated in

Table 6.1 Overview of individual and group-based approaches to cognitive training

Treatment	Description
Integrated Psychological Therapy (Brenner et al., 1980)	Integrated, group-based neurocognitive and social-cognitive training that focuses on improving cognitive differentiation, social perception, verbal communication, social skills, and interpersonal problem-solving
Cognitive Enhancement Therapy (Hogarty et al., 2004)	Developmental approach to cognitive remediation that integrates computer-based neurocognitive training in attention, memory, and problem-solving with group-based training in social cognition
Thinking Skills for Work (McGurk, 2005)	Integrated computerized cognitive remediation and individualized supported employment to address the neurocognitive factors that limit vocational functioning and to promote competitive employment
Social Cognition and Interaction Training (Penn et al., 2005)	Group-based social cognition training program that focuses on enhancing emotion perception, accurate causal attributions, and theory of mind
Neuropsychological Educational Approach to Remediation (Medalia, Revheim, & Herlands, 2009)	Eclectic and flexible group-based approach that integrates computerized neurocognitive training with bridging groups designed to promote the transfer of learned skills to everyday life
Social Cognitive Skills Training (Horan et al., 2009)	Group-based social cognition training program developed based on prior computerized and group-based approaches that focuses on improving emotion perception, social perception, theory of mind, and accurate causal attributions
Cognitive Remediation and Functional Adaptation Skills Training (Bowie et al., 2012)	Integrated computerized cognitive remediation with group-based behavioral skills training focused on improving medication management, social, and independent living skills

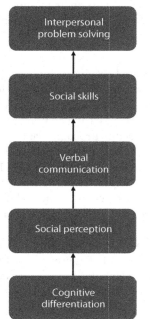

Figure 6.1 Hierarchical structure of Integrated Psychological Therapy (IPT) and its components

computerized programs are introduced to a small group of 5–7 patients, who work together to identify strategies that will enable the successful completion of the exercise. For example, patients may be given a series of index cards that require sorting based on a particular attribute, similar to the Wisconsin Card Sorting Test (Heaton et al., 1993), or word problems may be introduced, such as synonym or antonym exercises, to help patients develop understanding of broad conceptual categories. Group members work collaboratively to learn from each other, strategize over solutions, and build basic neurocognitive abilities.

The second component of IPT is social cognition training in social perception, or the ability to accurately recognize and encode social information. This component emphasizes distinguishing between relevant social information and environmental distractions that are not relevant for social understanding, and is delivered through 30–60 minute group-based training sessions. Similar to neurocognitive training, social perception training centers around solving cognitive exercises in the group, but in this case, exercises which are predominantly social in nature. For example, during the group sessions, patients are introduced to a social story through a series of slides, and asked to identify factual and observable information from these social scenes. As training progresses, the scenes contain more complex, ambiguous, and emotional information in them that require greater social perception ability to accurately characterize. Distinguishing fact from interpretation is a key strategy of focus during social perception training, as patients with schizophrenia have been repeatedly shown to "jump-to-conclusions," especially when stimuli are ambiguous (Moritz & Woodward, 2005; see Chapter 1). Individual interpretations of the social scenes are discussed as a whole group, with an emphasis on reality checking and avoiding interpretation beyond the available facts. In this way, patients learn to sharpen their social perception skills to identify relevant information in social situations without over-interpreting and drawing conclusions that are not consistent with reality.

After social perception training, IPT builds on the neurocognitive and social-cognitive abilities that have been learned thus far and begins to focus on improving verbal communication. IPT views neurocognitive and social perception training as necessary cognitive precursors to higher-order training in verbal communication, social skills, and problem-solving. In verbal communication training, patients focus on improving their attention toward speech from others and using reciprocity in conversations. Group exercises focus initially on attending to and repeating information presented during conversation, and then move to an emphasis on mutual communication between patients, where group members learn about the give-and-take in listening and speaking that characterizes reciprocal interpersonal interactions. Basic social skills training in asking appropriate questions to maintain a conversation are also taught to facilitate ongoing interaction and communication. Finally, the last two treatment components of IPT, social skills training, and interpersonal problem-solving, proceed to implement more traditional behavioral skills training interventions within a group modality. Social skills training relies on established methods from the schizophrenia treatment literature (Liberman et al., 1985; Wallace & Liberman, 1985), and builds on verbal communication skills to improve independent living, vocational, and interpersonal skills through behavioral rehearsal, observation, modeling, and role play. Interpersonal problem-solving training utilizes traditional problem-solving methods, but emphasizes cognitive analysis of different solutions and using knowledge of their success when applied to previous social situations.

The treatment components for IPT are delivered in a hierarchical, bottom-up fashion, such that neurocognitive training is expected to be introduced first to address attentional and other basic cognitive resources that will be needed for social perception and other training. Social perception training then comes after neurocognitive training to support training in verbal communication, social skills, and interpersonal problem-solving. These components are usually delivered over the course of 12–18 weeks, and because of its sequential and hierarchical nature, IPT is considered a bottom-up approach to cognitive remediation. A meta-analysis of over 25 years of research on IPT in schizophrenia indicated that this approach was associated with significant and medium-sized improvements in neurocognition, symptomatology, and psychosocial functioning (Roder, 2006).

6.3 Cognitive Enhancement Therapy (2004)

Cognitive Enhancement Therapy (Hogarty et al., 2004; Hogarty & Greenwald, 2006) is an 18-month, developmental approach to the remediation of social and non-social cognitive deficits that limit functional recovery from schizophrenia. The treatment was inspired by IPT, especially the early insights of Brenner and colleagues that recognized the power of a group modality and the significance of both neurocognitive and social-cognitive impairments in predicting functional disability. In CET, cognitive impairments related to schizophrenia are viewed as stemming from a neurodevelopmental insult resulting from the condition (Hogarty & Flesher, 1999; Keshavan, 1999), and the primary aim of CET is to "jump-start" cognitive development through providing enriched environmental and secondary socialization experiences. Hogarty and colleagues observed in the neuropsychological literature on schizophrenia that many of the performance characteristics of patients resembled those of healthy pre-adolescents. Individuals with the condition often process information in a serial manner, have difficulty selecting alternative problem-solving strategies, and do not consider the perspectives of others when navigating social situations. These are similar characteristics of pre-adolescent cognition, and Hogarty and colleagues hypothesized that the apparent developmental arrest associated with the condition could be improved through targeted cognitive exercises and secondary socialization experiences.

Over the course of 18 months, CET integrates 60 hours of computer-based training in attention, memory, and problem-solving with 45 structured social-cognitive group sessions. Neurocognitive training makes use of the Orientation Remedial Module (Ben-Yishay, Piasetsky, & Rattok, 1985) for attention training, and the PSSCogRehab suite (Bracy, 1994) is used for memory and problem-solving training (see Chapter 5 for a full description of these programs). Unlike most computerized cognitive enhancement approaches, neurocognitive training in CET is conducted in participant pairs and with the aid of a therapist/coach (see Figure 6.2). While one participant is working on a cognitive exercise, the second participant in the pair keeps score for her partner and provides support and encouragement during the training process. The pair of participants rotate between keeping score and completing a cognitive exercise throughout the 1-hour session. In the middle of the session, a 5-minute break is taken to relax and promote socialization among the two participants.

Therapist-coaches in neurocognitive training in CET introduce new cognitive exercises, set up the training exercise for the day, help participants think strategically about how to efficiently and effectively solve the problems presented by the exercise, and integrate concepts from the social-cognitive group into neurocognitive training. Because neurocognitive training during CET is performed in pairs with the aid of a coach, it resembles a small group. This structure has a number of significant advantages, as it offers many opportunities for socialization and the use of social cognition, enhances treatment

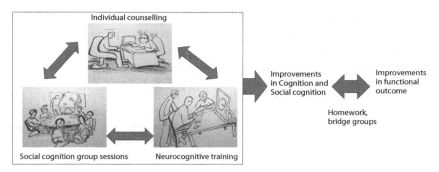

Figure 6.2 Integration of individual, computer, and group-based methods to cognitive enhancement

engagement and motivation, and builds familiarity between two patients and a coach who will ultimately be part of a larger social-cognitive group. There is also some evidence from our studies that a peer socialization component in the neurocognition training may benefit the enhancement of some aspects of cognition such as attention (Sandoval et al., 2017). The inclusion of a coach is also an innovation in computerized training that shifts training from a repetitive drill-and-practice approach to one that is more strategic in nature and promotes the acquisition of general cognitive abilities that can be applied to many different problems in everyday life beyond the given exercise. The coach is also essential for providing guidance and support, facilitating socialization among participants, and applying strategies learned in the social-cognitive group to neurocognitive training. Figure 6.2 illustrates the synergistic role of computer-based neurocognitive training, individual coaching sessions, and group sessions in facilitating cognitive enhancement.

Neurocognitive training in CET proceeds in a bottom-up, hierarchical fashion, similar to IPT. Attention and processing speed are the first targets of training and make use of exercises from the Orientation Remedial Module to enhance vigilance and rapid decision-making, inhibit irrelevant stimuli, and shift attention between auditory and visual modalities. Subsequent to attention training, the enhancement of memory focuses on developing a schematization or categorizing capacity, cognitive flexibility, an abstracting attitude, and executive (decision-making) functions using seven sequential, delayed, spatial, visual, auditory, and verbal memory routines that are contained in Bracy's PSSCogRehab suite. Strategy training is accomplished by helping patients develop a more gistful appreciation of abstract principles that underlie a working memory exercise, rather than a reliance on verbatim, declarative, or rote memory skills. Key CET concepts, such as internal coping, working memory, getting the gist, foresightfulness, and cognitive flexibility, introduced in the social cognitive group, are reinforced in memory training. Finally, problem-solving training incorporates discussion of the social-cognitive group curriculum and applications of key CET concepts (internal coping, gistfulness, foresightfulness, etc.) in performing various problem-solving computer tasks from Bracy's PSSCogRehab suite. Problem-solving training specifically targets analytic logic, effortful executive functions, strategic and foresightful planning. Together, these progressive neurocognitive activities are used to enhance basic information processing and support the developmental higher-order social-cognitive function through a seamless integration with the small-group, social cognition training component of CET.

After approximately 3 months of neurocognitive training in attention, 3–4 participant pairs and their coaches join to form a small social-cognitive group. These groups are the heart of the CET program and focus on the acquisition of adult social milestones in perspective-taking, social context appraisal, and other aspects of adult social cognition. There are a total of 45 1.5-hour social-cognitive group sessions that span three modules across the CET group curriculum, with each module containing relevant psychoeducational lectures, homework assignments and in-group exercises. The first module (Basic Concepts) introduces basic concepts about schizophrenia and its management, the role and regulation of stress in the disorder, the importance of medication, how to identify the main point or "gist" in communications, approaches to improving working memory and motivation, and ways to increase cognitive flexibility. The second module (Social Cognition) is directed toward the acquisition of key social-cognitive abilities (e.g. perspective-taking, foresightfulness, social context appraisal, recognition of emotion, and other non-verbal cues, giving support) and encourages patients to begin to utilize these principles in their everyday social interactions. The third module (CET Applications) focuses on the application and generalization of social-cognitive gains to everyday life, including interpersonal and vocational domains (see Table 6.2).

Each 1.5-hour social-cognitive group session is highly structured to contain predictable elements that serve to structure the group and help members become familiar and comfortable with its structure. In general, a typical session includes a Welcome Back to

Table 6.2 Cognitive Enhancement Therapy: illustration of an integrated computer- and group-based approach to cognitive remediation in schizophrenia

Component/Timeline[a]	Description
Neurocognitive training	
Attention training (months 0–4)	Computer-based exercises designed to improve processing speed, the ability to maintain a cognitive set, and sustained attention using the Orientation Remedial Module (Ben-Yishay, Piasetsky, & Rattok, 1985)
Memory training (months 5–11)	Computer-based exercises designed to improve working memory, strategic encoding of information, and use of compensatory memory aids using PSSCogRehab (Bracy, 1994)
Problem-solving training (months 12–18)	Computer-based exercises designed to improve planning, cognitive flexibility, and reasoning and logic using PSSCogRehab (Bracy, 1994)
Social-cognitive group curriculum	
Basic concepts (months 4–8)	Focuses on understanding and coping with schizophrenia, orientation to CET and components of CET, initial recovery plans, motivation, using gistful thinking, improving memory, and cognitive flexibility
Social cognition (months 9–14)	Focuses on acting wisely in social situations, social context appraisal, perspective-taking, reading non-verbal cues, emotional temperature taking, and other important aspects of social cognition
CET applications (months 15–18)	Focuses on generalizing CET to new situations, overcoming obstacles to using CET, and applying CET to respond to common social dilemmas, build social relationships, and initiate meaningful activities

Note. Adapted with permission from Eack (2013).
CET = Cognitive Enhancement Therapy.
[a]Timelines are approximate and intended to provide an illustration of the timing of treatment components delivered during CET.

introduce the agenda for the day; a Homework Presentation chaired by a group member to review and apply content learned in the previous week's psychoeducation lecture; a Cognitive Exercise that usually involves two group members; Feedback from all group members and coaches regarding performance on the exercise; a Psychoeducational lecture with summary handouts for each patient; and a New Homework Assignment for the next session, based on the lecture. In-group cognitive and social-cognitive exercises range from categorization exercises to using CET strategies to help a friend with a social problem to crafting gistful condensed messages that incorporate the perspectives of the sender and recipient of a message. Table 6.3 provides examples of these CET exercises (for more details see the CET manual by Hogarty and Greenwald (2006)).

Table 6.3 Selected example group exercises used in Cognitive Enhancement Therapy

Exercise	Description
Neurocognitive training	
Categorization	Sort words into categories; then re-sort the same set of words into a new set of categories.
Soundbyte	Extract the main point (gist) and minor points from newspaper opinion editorials. Take the author's perspective and Engage? in a debate about the pro and con side of the issue.
Introduce yourself	Give a brief presentation on yourself to the group, using a structured outline describing the qualities you value in yourself.
Condensed message	Send a brief, gistful message to a receiver that will get him or her to act in an intended way.
Using CET to help a friend	Respond to a friend who is having challenge with social cognition using strategies learned in CET.

Note. See Hogarty and Greenwald (2006) for full description of all exercises used in CET.

Case Study 6.1

Michael is a 30-year-old former college student who has been struggling to get back to school after having developed schizophrenia while away at college. Jay is a 25-year-old who developed schizoaffective disorder after high school and desperately wants to make more friends. Both have considerable interpersonal challenges. Michael has trouble organizing what he wants to say in conversations and remembering the topic of discussion. Jay is very shy and has almost completely withdrawn socially after the onset of his condition. This week in CET, it is their turn to work together on the in-group social-cognitive exercise, Condensed Message. In this week's Condensed Message called "The Airport," Michael and Jay read a social scenario where a son is dropping his father off at the airport. They have a little time and decide to get something to eat at one of the airport restaurants. On his route home, the son receives a call from the airport restaurant telling him that his father has forgotten his wallet there. The airport is very busy, and the restaurant offers to send a page announcement throughout the airport notifying the father that he needs to pick up his wallet before boarding his flight. Since the announcement is sent over the public address system, it needs to be brief, and the son needs to construct a ten-word message that will get his father to act quickly before his flight leaves.

After Michael and Jay read the scenario together, they move to the front of the group and draw ten lines ("____ ____ ...") on the whiteboard. The coach in the group explains that their first task is to identify the problem presented in the scenario. The team works together for a minute, and Michael blurts out, "He's gotta give his dad his wallet!" Jay agrees, but the coach questions, "Does the son need to give his dad the wallet directly?" Jay is looking down and is somewhat disengaged. Michael affirms, "Yes!" The coach then asks Jay, "Do you agree?" Jay lifts his head and says, "He needs to tell his dad to go get the wallet". "Excellent!", the coach replies, and confirms that the problem is that the son needs to send a message to the father to get his wallet. The coach then explains that their next task is to identify the perspectives of the sender and recipient of the message. "Who is the sender and who is the receiver of the message in this situation?", the coach asks. Jay indicates that the son needs to send the message to his father. "And what is the son's perspective in this situation?", asks the coach. Michael indicates, "Jay just said, he needs to send a message to his father!" "Very true", the coach indicates, "But what might he be thinking and feeling?" The team is a bit stumped by the question, obviously struggling to understand the son's perspective. Michael says, "He's probably worried - what if his father doesn't have any money for his trip?" "Excellent!", the coach says, providing positive rein-forcement. The coach then reminds the team to work together and for Michael to check in with his partner, Jay, on what he thinks the son's perspective might be. Jay struggles more, and the coach asks, "What does the son want to convey in his message? What does he want out of this situation?" Jay lights up, "He wants his father to go back to the restaurant to get his wallet!" "Exactly", the coach replies. Having figured out the son's perspective, the team moves on to discuss the father's point of view and what he might need to hear in a brief message in order to return to the restaurant before his flight leaves.

Now that the team has figured out the problem to be addressed and the perspectives of the sender and recipient of the message, it is time to start crafting the ten-word page to be sent over the intercom. Michael, often being the first to speak, delivers a long and convoluted message well beyond the ten-word limit. The coach refrains from intervening, and asks him to check out his ideas with his partner. Jay says, "Well, that sounds good, but it's a little long." Michael rushes to the whiteboard and attempts to write down his state-ment in the space provided, and ultimately realizes that this is going to be harder than it looks. He attempts to come up with a second statement, but it is even longer and less focused.

The coach asks Jay, "What do you think?" Jay makes the important point, "Well, we need to start by saying the name of the person the message is for." "OK, Michael go ahead and erase what you have started, and listen to Jay, he has a good point", the coach replies. Michael agrees and they start the statement with the father's name, "Dr. McIsaacs." Michael adds to this and says, "Pick up your wallet at the restaurant immediately before you board your flight." The coach asks, "How long is that statement?" Jay and Michael agree that it is too long, and they shorten it to "Dr. McIsaacs pick up your wallet at the restaurant immediately."

The coach then asks the participants to consider whether they should announce to the whole airport that a wallet is available. Like many patients with schizophrenia-spectrum conditions, Jay and Michael have ignored the social context of a busy airport with many people who might be interested in such a wallet. The participants have also overlooked the fact that airports typically have many restaurants, and more information is needed as to the specific restaurant holding the lost item. With some teamwork and coaching, Michael and Jay refine their message to "Dr. McIsaacs get lost item at Blue Angel restaurant immediately" and successfully solve the exercise. They receive a round of applause from the group, and then the non-participating group members and coaches provide feedback on their handling of the intellectual, emotional, and social challenges of the exercise.

These exercises usually involve two group members, while the remaining members observe and prepare structured feedback on exercise performance. The above case examples of Michael and Jay (see case study) illustrate the process of social cognition training using in-group exercises and the integrated nature of social-cognitive training in CET, where numerous abilities are targeted within a single exercise surrounding a real-world social situation. In this particular exercise, perspective-taking is essential for crafting a message that will address the problem and get the recipient to act accordingly, but so are social context appraisal and gistfulness in developing the brief message. Teamwork is also essential, and like many other CET exercises, Condensed Message provides ample opportunity to practice working as a team, performing in front of a group, and managing stress and social anxiety associated with participating in the exercise.

Beyond neurocognitive and social-cognitive training, CET also makes use of individual sessions through weekly one-on-one meetings between the patient and coach to personalize the treatment to his or her particular goals. The coach works with patients to identify goals related to cognitive enhancement and link broader functional goals to cognitive challenges they are experiencing, such as difficulties with attention and problems completing classes for school. These goals are formulated into a recovery plan that identifies the primary goal, problem, and set of strategies to be learned and applied during CET to help patients achieve their goals. In this manner, although CET is a group-based treatment, each patient has a personalized approach to rehabilitation that is tailored to their specific needs and goals.

The efficacy of CET has been demonstrated across clinical trials of chronic (Hogarty et al., 2004) and early course patients with schizophrenia (Eack et al., 2009), and the program has been recognized by the United States government as an evidence-based practice (www.legacy.nreppadmin.net/ViewIntervention.aspx?id=273). CET is associated with medium-to-large improvements in both neurocognitive and social-cognitive outcomes, as well as significant improvements in functioning (see Figure 6.3).

Early course schizophrenia patients treated with CET were more likely to obtain competitive employment than those not treated with CET (54% vs. 18%) in a recent controlled trial (Eack et al., 2010). Although most trials have excluded individuals with comorbid addiction problems, a recent study showed that CET was feasible and potentially effective for patients with schizophrenia with comorbid cannabis and/or alcohol use problems (Eack et al., 2015). Finally, the early application of CET has been shown to be neuroprotective, preventing both gray matter loss (Eack et al., 2010) and strengthening prefrontal cortical networks (Keshavan et al., 2017) associated with cognitive impairment in schizophrenia, highlighting the neurobiological mechanisms by which this intervention achieves its pro-cognitive effects.

6.4 Social Cognition and Interaction Training (2005)

Social Cognition and Interaction Training (SCIT; Penn et al., 2005) is another group-based social cognition training program that focuses on improving emotion perception, causal attributions, and theory of mind, the three areas of social cognition that have repeatedly shown impairment in patients with schizophrenia (Green et al., 2008; Penn et al., 1997). Like CET, SCIT is manual-driven and group sessions are highly structured, with an introductory "Check-In," followed by homework review, an in-group social-cognitive exercise,

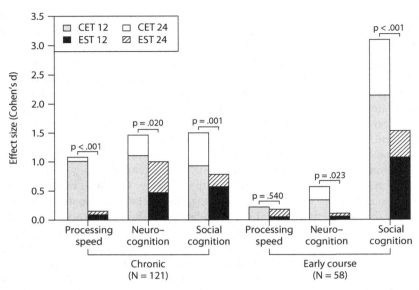

Figure 6.3 Effect sizes of Cognitive Enhancement Therapy in chronic and early course schizophrenia Adapted from Hogarty et al. (2004). *Archives of General Psychiatry, 61*(9), 866–876 and Eack et al. (2009). *Psychiatric Services, 60*(11), 1468–1476.

and then a homework assignment to facilitate application (Roberts & Penn, 2009). Group sessions are typically conducted weekly for 50 minutes over the course of 18–24 weeks. Social-cognitive exercises performed in the group are designed to develop knowledge around a particularly relevant aspect of social cognition (e.g. jumping to conclusions) and strengthen that ability through practice and observation. These exercises most often consist of analyzing social stimuli to enhance detection of relevant and accurate information, such as identifying and defining emotions in faces or making mental inferences from social scenarios. Video demonstrations of faux pas are also used as a method of learning about various aspects of social cognition and the interpersonal consequences of social-cognitive fallacies, with use of the HBO Special Curb Your Enthusiasm with Larry David as a particularly innovative example (Ward, 2007). Other exercises are more problem-solving in nature, and ask participants to identify challenging social situations, to which the group therapist guides the patient through a social analysis of the situation (e.g. identifying the feelings of people involved, distinguishing facts from inferences) and possible alternative solutions.

Over the course of the treatment, SCIT contains three distinct phases that focus on emotion training, figuring out situations, and integration, respectively. Emotion training teaches patients about the different basic emotions, how to identify them in faces, and how they influence and are influenced by social situations. These skills are taught using visual aids (e.g. pictures of people) and didactic instruction, and patients are also introduced to computer-based methods of emotion perception training, such as those reviewed in Chapter 5. However, SCIT extends beyond traditional emotion perception training to also introduce the concept of suspiciousness and how patients can use social cues and avoid jumping to conclusions to identify warranted and unwarranted suspiciousness.

The second phase of SCIT, figuring out situations, aims to address cognitive inflexibility, jumping-to-conclusions, and other aspects of dysfunctional attributional style that are characteristic of schizophrenia. Group members become sensitive to the distinction between facts and "social guesses" and work with the therapists to interpret ambiguous situations factually and avoid premature conclusions. In one exercise, patients are asked to independently generate a list of facts and guesses from a photograph and then compare their list to other members of the group, which highlights variability in what is perceived as factual, as well as the commonalities in what was perceived that justify the selection of facts from the picture. Another exercise is similar to the game 20 questions, where points are rewarded the more questions that are asked, in an effort to reduce jumping-to-conclusions and help patients increase their tolerance of ambiguity.

The final phase of SCIT is integration, which focuses on application of learned skills and abilities from the group to everyday life. Real social problems from outside the group are introduced by group members, and then the group proceeds to analyze that problem and determine solutions based on identifying the emotions present, determining fact from guess, avoiding jumping to conclusions, and understanding the social situation. In the case of uncertainty, patients can "check it out" by asking other group members, the therapist, or people in the actual situation. Role-plays are also used to help practice responses and possible outcomes from the different solutions generated. Care is taken to ensure that all group members are involved in the problem-solving process, even if they did not raise the social problem or it does not personally apply to them, so that members get an opportunity to practice applying social-cognitive abilities learned in SCIT.

The efficacy of SCIT for improving social cognition and functioning has been evaluated in several initial controlled trials with schizophrenia inpatients and outpatients. In an inpatient study of 28 patients with schizophrenia, Combs and colleagues (2007) found that patients treated with SCIT showed significant improvements in emotion perception, theory of mind, attributional style, and cognitive flexibility compared to/with a coping skills comparison condition. A study of 31 outpatients with schizophrenia showed significant improvements in emotion perception and social skills using performance-based assessments. However, effects on theory of mind and attributional style were not significant, as previously observed in the inpatient study. A recent randomized-controlled trial of 66 outpatients with schizophrenia replicated previously observed beneficial effects on emotion perception, social skill, and attributional style. Further, some benefits were observed favoring SCIT on measures of symptomatology, particularly negative symptoms and general psychopathology. Evidence of functional improvement from SCIT has been more limited, although these prior trials have shown significant gains in social skill and long-term follow-up may be needed to identify effects on broader domains of functioning.

6.5 Neuropsychological Educational Approach to Remediation (2009)

The Neuropsychological Educational Approach to Remediation (NEAR) is an eclectic, individualized cognitive remediation intervention developed for patients with a variety of psychiatric conditions, including schizophrenia (Medalia, Revheim, & Casey, 2002; Medalia et al., 2009). The approach is entirely group-based, and provides both computerized-cognitive training and group-based "bridging" of cognitive skills to everyday functional outcomes within a flexible curriculum. Computerized training takes place in a group setting where 3–9 patients gather at a set of computer workstations to complete various cognitive exercises facilitated by a clinician. Unlike most other computer- and group-based cognitive remediation approaches, NEAR does not prescribe a specific set of computer programs to be used during rehabilitation, but rather, makes use of relevant commercially available software programs that would be beneficial for the patient. In order to be utilized in the NEAR approach, computerized routines must be engaging and target neuropsychological deficits, and NEAR is unique in that it allows for an evolving field of computerized approaches to cognitive remediation. Given that many software programs now exist for enhancing cognition across a variety of populations, the use of an open curriculum in computerized training has clear advantages and allows NEAR to utilize the latest available software for targeting neurocognitive impairments.

Cognitive training is built around a three-stage curriculum, focused on basic, intermediate, and advanced cognitive skills. In the basic phase, lower order abilities in attention or working memory are targeted using relatively low difficulty settings that are achievable by even more impaired patients. This phase introduces the value of cognitive remediation to patients and prepares them for more advanced, higher-order training. In the intermediate phase, task difficulty is increased and cognitive exercises begin to address abilities that are more complex and, at times, distal from immediate goals (e.g. concept formation). In the final, advanced phase higher-order cognitive abilities are addressed in complex problem-solving and other domains, and cognitive exercises frequently rely on multiple cognitive abilities. Task demands are high, as is task difficulty, and goals for the exercise may require multiple sessions to complete. These three phases represent NEAR "Building Blocks", which are used to develop treatment plans and guide the progress of computerized training throughout the course of intervention (Medalia et al., 2009). Continuing its individualized and flexible perspective on treatment, NEAR allows patients to move through these three building blocks of cognitive enhancement at their own pace, based on their strengths and needs, leading to a phased approach to cognitive remediation that is pragmatic, adaptable to many settings, and capable of being tailored to a wide patient population.

The computerized training component of NEAR is integrated with *bridging groups* to facilitate the translation of learned cognitive abilities to functional improvement in everyday life. These bridging groups consist of a small number of patients and use discussion and in-group exercises to link cognitive abilities to functional goals, practice learned skills, and prepare for their generalization outside of the clinical setting. Specific cognitive abilities are discussed, such as attention, and their importance for various aspects of daily life to help patients understand the functional significance of the skills they are learning. Motivation is facilitated using this and other approaches, and Medalia and colleagues have been pioneers in incorporating methods to enhance motivation in their treatment approach (Choi & Medalia, 2010; Medalia & Saperstein, 2011). In-group exercises also provide opportunities to practice cognitive skills and their application to common real-world scenarios, such as cooking, creating a calendar, and maintaining a schedule. These exercises are organized as group projects that have a larger functional goal (e.g. organizing a pot-luck dinner) and require multiple cognitive abilities to complete, such as attention, planning, and problem-solving. Some discussion of the impact of neurocognitive abilities on interpersonal and social abilities is also covered, although the approach does not specifically target social cognition.

Quite unique to NEAR is the use of peer leaders during the course of computerized training and bridging groups. Peers are those patients who have been involved in NEAR for a longer period of time and have developed some mastery and expertise with the intervention. Because both neurocognitive training and bridging groups have rolling admissions, there are naturally some individuals involved in these activities with greater experience than others. In some cases, these individuals become peer leaders and share their learning with newcomers, serve as an example of the benefits of cognitive remediation, and provide mentorship to their peers about illness management and functional recovery. The use of peer leaders not only facilitates motivation and engagement among newer members of the treatment, but also helps to build self-confidence and social skills among the peer leaders.

Several studies have been conducted evaluating the efficacy of NEAR in patients with schizophrenia and other severe mental illnesses, although a number of these studies have been small in size and have not been published in the peer-reviewed literature (Medalia & Freilich, 2008). Effects on cognition have been primarily observed in the domains of attention and processing speed (Choi & Medalia, 2005; Medalia, Herlands, & Baginsky, 2003). Studies of the effects of NEAR on functional outcomes have found significant improvements in readiness for clerical work and work-related behavior (Choi & Medalia, 2005). Further, another uncontrolled study with homeless individuals with severe mental illness found significant improvements in enrollment in educational programs and vocational internships (Medalia et al., 2003). Although the rigor of the evidence base for NEAR is at times limited, the flexibility of the program has resulted in its widespread implementation throughout various research studies (Keefe et al., 2012) and community agencies.

6.6 Social Cognitive Skills Training (2009)

Another group-based approach that focuses not only on neuropsychological rehabilitation, but also on social cognition training is Social-Cognitive Skills Training, a 6- to 24-week small-group approach designed to improve emotion perception, theory of mind, social perception, and correct attribution of intentionality and events (Horan et al., 2009). This approach builds on Penn and Robert's SCIT intervention, as well as an emotion perception training program by Frommann, Streit, and Wölwer (2003), and was developed by Horan, Green, and other colleagues from the University of California, Los Angeles, who have led landmark studies of neurocognitive and social-cognitive dysfunction in schizophrenia.

Social-Cognitive Skills Training is also a phased/modularized approach, with the first phase focusing on emotion and social perception training. Participants receive psychoeducation on the basic emotions and contexts in which they are produced, as well as detecting emotional prosody in speech. Computer aids are used to demonstrate emotions in faces and speech, and the emotion perception computer training exercises of Wölwer and colleagues (Wölwer, Frommann, & Halfmann, 2005) are employed to provide training in the identification of facial emotions. Subsequently, training is provided in social cue perception and social context appraisal using novel materials providing education on social norms and non-verbal gestures outside of facial affect. Further, the influence of emotion on thinking and behavior in social situations is also discussed, and digital photos and movie clips are used to aid instruction on these concepts. The second phase of Social-Cognitive Skills Training focuses on theory of mind and address attributional biases, particularly jumping-to-conclusions (Moritz & Woodward, 2005). In-group exercises and materials are presented to improve the ability of patients to understand the intentions of others, identify how paranoia may impair that understanding, and to help patients learn how to test for evidence of their beliefs, similar to approaches employed in cognitive behavioral therapy for psychosis (Kingdon & Turkington, 1994).

Several randomized-controlled trials have been conducted on Social Cognitive Skills Training in outpatients with schizophrenia. The strongest effects appear to be on facial emotion perception (Horan et al., 2009) and emotion management (Horan et al., 2011), two domains of social cognition that are significantly impaired in this condition (Green et al., 2008). Effects on functional outcome have not been described in these trials, although significant improvements in social skill have been observed at treatment completion (Horan et al., 2011). A recent 6-week randomized trial found that when Social Cognitive Skills Training was provided in conjunction with oxytocin, patients with schizophrenia showed significant increases in empathic accuracy (Davis et al., 2014). These findings indicate that Social Cognitive Skills Training can produce significant improvements in various domains of emotion processing, either alone or when combined with other forms of cognitive treatment.

6.7 Integrated Models

There are numerous cognitive remediation models that are designed to be integrated within larger psychosocial rehabilitation and other group-based intervention programs for people living with schizophrenia (see Figure 6.2). Perhaps the most well-studied of these models is McGurk's Thinking Skills for Work program, which embeds computerized training with Cogpak (see Chapter 5) and other cognitive remediation interventions with supported employment. This approach utilizes neurocognitive training and takes a strategic training approach to help participants learn to more effectively solve problems and accomplish tasks in cognitive exercises. In addition, compensatory training is provided to help patients cope with persistent cognitive challenges. Short- and long-term effects of Thinking Skills for Work have demonstrated marked improvements in competitive employment in people living with schizophrenia (McGurk, 2005; McGurk et al., 2007). A recent trial with patients who were treatment-resistant to traditional supported employment has also indicated that Thinking Skills for Work can produce a near two-fold increase in the percentage of patients who are able to obtain competitive jobs (McGurk et al., 2015). The studies of McGurk and colleagues are also particularly notable for their frequent inclusion of those with substance use comorbidity and greater proportion of those with an ethnic or racial minority background, providing more generalizable data than is often obtained in clinical trials of cognitive remediation interventions.

Another integrated cognitive remediation approach comes from the work of Bowie and colleagues, who have combined a group-based psychosocial intervention, functional adaptation skills training, with computer-based cognitive remediation. In this approach, Bowie and colleagues (Bowie et al., 2012) provided 12 weeks of computer-based cognitive remediation based on the Thinking Skills for Work program, and then participants received 12 weeks of functional adaptation skills training. The later approach was originally developed for older patients with schizophrenia (Patterson et al., 2003), and employs a structured group format that provides skills training social and independent living skills, such as transportation, finances, and medication management. Functional adaptation skills training uses a highly structured group curriculum that consists of psychoeducation, homework, and in-session practice and behavioral modeling using role-plays. Bowie and colleagues have conducted a randomized-controlled trial of cognitive remediation, functional adaptation skills training, or their combination in outpatients with schizophrenia (Bowie et al., 2012). These investigators found that significant functional improvements were only observed in individuals who received combined cognitive remediation and functional adaptation skills training, which is congruent with previous meta-analytic evidence indicating greater improvements in functional outcome when cognitive remediation interventions are integrated within larger psychosocial rehabilitation programs (McGurk et al., 2007). Such studies should serve to remind readers that the treatments that surround cognitive remediation are as important as the cognitive remediation intervention itself, and that to promote functional recovery in schizophrenia, multi-element interventions are likely to be necessary.

6.8 Evidence Base for Cognitive Enhancement in Schizophrenia

This chapter, along with Chapter 5 on computer-based approaches to cognitive training, has presented the broad landscape of cognitive remediation options for schizophrenia that have been evaluated in the scientific literature. All of the approaches to cognitive enhancement reviewed have at least a minimal evidence base, and some approaches, such as Posit Science, CET, and Thinking Skills for Work have been evaluated in multiple randomized-controlled trials demonstrating their efficacy. But what about the overall impact of cognitive enhancement approaches, generally, for patients with schizophrenia and related disorders? An early meta-analytic review by McGurk and colleagues (McGurk et al., 2007) showed that as an eclectic set of approaches, cognitive enhancement can significantly improve cognitive and functional outcomes in schizophrenia, particularly when embedded within larger psychosocial rehabilitation programs, such as supported employment or social cognition training. An updated meta-analysis was conducted by Wykes and colleagues in 2011 continuing to demonstrate the efficacy of computer-, individual-, and group-based approaches to cognitive enhancement (Wykes et al., 2011; see also Chapters 8 and 9). Effect sizes for each study are presented in Figure 6.4.

While there is considerable heterogeneity in effect sizes across studies, on average the authors of the review found that cognitive enhancement in schizophrenia was associated with significant improvements in cognition ($d = 0.45$), functioning ($d = 0.42$), and symptomatology ($d = 0.18$), although effects on symptoms were small. Interestingly, the authors found that the methodological quality of the study did not impact the resulting effect size of cognitive training. However, similar to the observations of McGurk and colleagues, provision of strategic training and adjunctive psychosocial rehabilitation in the context of cognitive training significantly improved effects on functioning. Further, patients who presented with less symptomatology were more likely to experience a greater cognitive benefit associated with treatment (Wykes et al., 2011).

With regard to social-cognitive training, specifically, Kurtz and Richardson (2011) conducted a comprehensive meta-analysis of 19 controlled trials in schizophrenia. The approaches reviewed represented diverse methods of social-cognitive enhancement, from computer-based approaches to group-based models. The authors found that social cognition training was associated with significant improvements in emotion perception ($d = 0.71$) and theory of mind ($d = 0.46$), as well as improved functional outcome ($d = 0.78$). Impact on social cue perception and attributional style was non-significant, likely due to the limited number of studies that have addressed this domain during

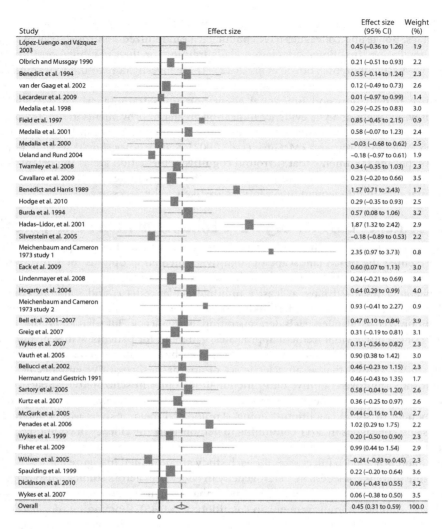

Study	Effect size	Effect size (95% CI)	Weight (%)
López-Luengo and Vázquez 2003		0.45 (–0.36 to 1.26)	1.9
Olbrich and Mussgay 1990		0.21 (–0.51 to 0.93)	2.2
Benedict et al. 1994		0.55 (–0.14 to 1.24)	2.3
van der Gaag et al. 2002		0.12 (–0.49 to 0.73)	2.6
Lecardeur et al. 2009		0.01 (–0.97 to 0.99)	1.4
Medalia et al. 1998		0.29 (–0.25 to 0.83)	3.0
Field et al. 1997		0.85 (–0.45 to 2.15)	0.9
Medalia et al. 2001		0.58 (–0.07 to 1.23)	2.4
Medalia et al. 2000		–0.03 (–0.68 to 0.62)	2.5
Ueland and Rund 2004		–0.18 (–0.97 to 0.61)	1.9
Twamley et al. 2008		0.34 (–0.35 to 1.03)	2.3
Cavallaro et al. 2009		0.23 (–0.20 to 0.66)	3.5
Benedict and Harris 1989		1.57 (0.71 to 2.43)	1.7
Hodge et al. 2010		0.29 (–0.35 to 0.93)	2.5
Burda et al. 1994		0.57 (0.08 to 1.06)	3.2
Hadas–Lidor, et al. 2001		1.87 (1.32 to 2.42)	2.9
Silverstein et al. 2005		–0.18 (–0.89 to 0.53)	2.2
Meichenbaum and Cameron 1973 study 1		2.35 (0.97 to 3.73)	0.8
Eack et al. 2009		0.60 (0.07 to 1.13)	3.0
Lindenmayer et al. 2008		0.24 (–0.21 to 0.69)	3.4
Hogarty et al. 2004		0.64 (0.29 to 0.99)	4.0
Meichenbaum and Cameron 1973 study 2		0.93 (–0.41 to 2.27)	0.9
Bell et al. 2001–2007		0.47 (0.10 to 0.84)	3.9
Greig et al. 2007		0.31 (–0.19 to 0.81)	3.1
Wykes et al. 2007		0.13 (–0.56 to 0.82)	2.3
Vauth et al. 2005		0.90 (0.38 to 1.42)	3.0
Bellucci et al. 2002		0.46 (–0.23 to 1.15)	2.3
Hermanutz and Gestrich 1991		0.46 (–0.43 to 1.35)	1.7
Sartory et al. 2005		0.58 (–0.04 to 1.20)	2.6
Kurtz et al. 2007		0.36 (–0.25 to 0.97)	2.6
McGurk et al. 2005		0.44 (–0.16 to 1.04)	2.7
Penades et al. 2006		1.02 (0.29 to 1.75)	2.2
Wykes et al. 1999		0.20 (–0.50 to 0.90)	2.3
Fisher et al. 2009		0.99 (0.44 to 1.54)	2.9
Wölwer et al. 2005		–0.24 (–0.93 to 0.45)	2.3
Spaulding et al. 1999		0.22 (–0.20 to 0.64)	3.6
Dickinson et al. 2010		0.06 (–0.43 to 0.55)	3.2
Wykes et al. 2007		0.06 (–0.38 to 0.50)	3.5
Overall		0.45 (0.31 to 0.59)	100.0

0

Figure 6.4 Effect sizes from a meta-analytic review of cognitive enhancement approaches in schizophrenia
Reprinted with permission from Wykes et al. (2011), *American Journal of Psychiatry, 168*(5), 472–485.

treatment. A number of moderators were also found of treatment efficacy, particularly that younger patients tended to show greater functional improvement associated with social-cognitive training.

Overall, the findings from these meta-analytic reviews indicate that cognitive enhancement is a robust evidence-based practice that is supported by a mature and diverse scientific literature. There are now over 40 randomized-controlled trials of cognitive training in patients with schizophrenia, and while there are many differences between approaches, on average their efficacy is well-supported and suggests that the treatment of cognition using these approaches is an important avenue for supporting functional recovery in patients with schizophrenia and related disorders.

6.9 Choosing Among Various Approaches to Cognitive Enhancement

The wide range of available computer-based, individual and group-based approaches to cognitive enhancement as outlined in this and the previous chapter raises the question for the clinician as to which programs to choose for a given patient on a given clinical setting. While in this volume we have focused somewhat more prominently on our own approach, CET, we believe that there are strengths and weaknesses to each program and the choice is best made on a case-by-case basis for each individual situation, keeping in mind the key principles underlying successful outcome with cognitive enhancement interventions as outlined in Chapter 3. In other words, it is likely that there is not a single menu that is ideal for all patients and a greater description of how to select the right treatment for the right patient is discussed in Chapter 10.

6.10 Summary

- There exist numerous options for individual and group-based cognitive training in patients with schizophrenia and a significant evidence base is emerging supporting their efficacy for improving cognition and functioning.
- Many group-based interventions focus on social cognition and the group context appears to be a powerful tool for enhancing social-cognitive outcomes.
- Individual and group therapy sessions can be effective contexts to personalize and practice the abilities gained in computerized cognitive training, and some use these contexts to create a bridge between cognitive improvement and functional recovery.
- Some of the most robust effects of cognitive remediation on functional outcomes in schizophrenia have come from intervention models that integrate computerized training with individual and small-group approaches, as well as rehabilitative approaches such as supported employment.
- Cognitive enhancement is an evidence-based practice in schizophrenia that is supported by a large number of scientific studies. The informed clinician has a wide range of cognitive enhancement approaches from which to choose.

Psychopharmacological Approaches, Cognitive Enhancement, and Brain Stimulation

Symptomatic stabilization by optimal use of antipsychotics and other psychotropic medication is a critical precondition for the success of cognitive enhancement interventions. In this chapter, we will review the psychopharmacological treatment of psychotic disorders first. We will then briefly summarize our knowledge about the pharmacological agents, neuromodulation and other approaches that have been investigated for their potential efficacy in improving cognition.

7.1 Pharmacotherapy of Psychotic Disorders

Antipsychotic drugs are the mainstay in the pharmacological treatment of psychotic disorders. Several considerations are important to keep in mind, which may be summarized as the ten "commandments" of pharmacotherapy (Box 7.1). A detailed description of the approaches to psychopharmacology of psychotic disorders is beyond the scope of this chapter, and the reader is referred to more detailed reviews of this topic (Tandon, Nasrallah, & Keshavan, 2010).

Connecting and Consent

The importance of "joining" in a positive therapeutic alliance has already been discussed in Chapter 4. Given the risk of significant side effects (such as metabolic side effects and tardive dyskinesia) with antipsychotic and other medications used to treat schizophrenia and related disorders, it is important that the benefits and risks of medications be discussed with patients early in treatment, at an appropriate time. Informed consent and education are critically important. Informed consent is not a one-time task, but is an interactive process that should occur with many opportunities for questions.

Comprehensive Assessment and Care

Unfortunately, with the progressive fragmentation of psychiatric care in recent years, managed care pressures and decreasing reimbursements, pharmacotherapy and psychotherapy are rarely if ever conducted by the same treating clinician; for psychiatrists, the "15-minute med check" has become the norm, though it robs patients of the opportunity for integrated care management. For optimum success, it is critical for the psychiatrist and the therapist to be "on the same page" and preferably be part of the same team to avoid the problem of "split care."

Box 7.1 The key principles to consider in pharmacotherapy of psychotic disorders

Connecting and consent

Comprehensive assessment

Collaborative (shared) decision-making

Comprehensive care

Choice of the medication(s)

Correct dose and duration

Ensuring compliance

Addressing comorbidity

Continuity of care

Managing side effects

Managing treatment resistance

Collaborative Care

There is some evidence that shared decision-making improves treatment outcomes (Stovell et al., 2016). It is especially valuable for patients who have reasonable decisional capacity (Hamann et al., 2009) and a good therapeutic alliance. Even patients who dislike their medications often benefit from some autonomy afforded to make some choices, such as the type of medication, and the dose. Some of the most effective medication decisions are collaborative ones, and research has increasingly indicated the importance of shared decision-making in medication adherence and outcomes in people with schizophrenia (Deegan & Drake, 2006). Pharmacological (and non-pharmacological) treatments are most effective when they are grounded in a shared decision-making approach. At every visit, the clinician should inquire about the patient's satisfaction with the medications, and whether he/she thinks any change needs to be made.

Most of the time, discussions will pertain to the questions of which medication(s) to take, and about how to minimize side effects and enhance efficacy. A larger challenge arises when the question involves whether to take medication at all. Relapse prevention studies in general support the importance of continued medications, except in a small proportion of patients who may do well despite no medications. However, at this time, we have no good way to predict who might have such a favorable outcome.

A dialogue with patients on this question would benefit from (a) a review of available data on relapse frequencies; (b) involving the family in the decision making process; (c) very gradual dose reduction to the point of minimum effective dose, which may be acceptable to many patients; (d) developing an agreement with the patient for continued treatment for a specified minimum length of time, with an option to revisit the decision periodically; and finally, (e) in selected cases, very gradual discontinuation with education, early detection of relapse, and contingency plans to reinstitute medication as quickly as possible. It is important to maintain the therapeutic relationship during periods of non-compliance.

Choice of Antipsychotic

Most antipsychotics, with the possible exception of clozapine, have subtle, if any, differences in efficacy. There is some evidence, however, that atypical antipsychotics have some advantages over first generation (or "typical") antipsychotics in first episode patients, though this is to be tempered by the higher prevalence of weight gain and metabolic side effects (Zhang et al., 2013). Atypical, or second-generation antipsychotics have a lower propensity to cause extrapyramidal side effects such as Parkinsonism and dystonia. They owe their advantage to the fact that they produce their antipsychotic effects at a lower degree of dopaminergic blockade (Figure 7.1). It is, therefore, common to choose an antipsychotic drug based on side effects the clinician and the patient wish to *avoid* (Table 7.1); other considerations include previous treatment response, patient preference, route and frequency of administration, and cost.

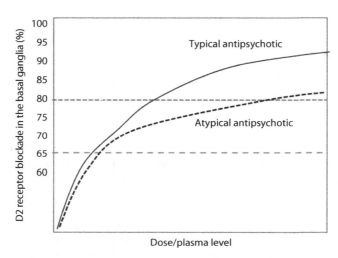

Figure 7.1 The key difference between first and second generation antipsychotics lies in the former (solid line) producing higher levels of D2 receptor blockade causing extrapyramidal side effects at therapeutic doses. Atypical antipsychotics produce their therapeutic effects with lower levels of D2 blockade

Table 7.1 Advantages and disadvantages of antipsychotic drug

	Advantages	**Disadvantages**
First generation APDs (e.g. haloperidol, fluphenazine, thiothixene, perphenazine, chlorpromazine, trifluperazine)	Effective with positive symptoms Relatively low risk of weight gain/ metabolic syndrome Haloperidol useful in delirium, pregnancy	Extrapyramidal syndromes (EPS) such as Parkinsonism and akathisia Prolactin elevation, sexual dysfunction
Atypical Second generation APDs (aripiprazole, clozapine, olanzapine, quetiapine, risperidone, iloperidone, ziprasidone, lurasidone, asenapine, cariprazine, brexpiprazole)	Effective with positive symptoms, Relatively low EPS potential[a] Relatively less prolactin elevation[b]	Weight gain[c] Increased risk of metabolic syndrome (though not all atypical APDs) Expensive

[a]Risperidone at higher doses induces EPS with greater frequency.
[b]Risperidone tends to increase prolactin levels.
[c]Greatest weight gain is seen with clozapine and olanzapine.

Treatment resistance is common, and can be seen in about a third of patients. Treatment resistance is often the result of the wrong diagnosis, non-adherence to medications, comorbid conditions, or inadequate blood levels due to pharmacokinetic (e.g. excessive smoking can reduce antipsychotic blood levels) or pharmacogenetic reasons (e.g. poor treatment response in rapid metabolizers). Clozapine is effective in treating some patients with treatment resistance, and should be considered early in treatment.

Correct Dose and Duration

Most patients respond to 300–700 mg chlorpromazine equivalents (relative potency of APDs compared to a standard dose of chlorpromazine). First episode patients may respond to doses that are 50–60% of those used in chronic patients (Robinson et al., 2015). However, when initiating treatment, it is good to *Start Low, Go Slow*. The aim of treatment is to arrive at maximal therapeutic benefit using the lowest effective dose while minimizing side effects. This is best achieved with a "minimum effective dose" approach. Decreasing the likelihood of side effects will enhance treatment adherence, which will, in turn improve treatment response.

The key questions faced by the clinician, and often asked by patients and family members alike are: How long should one continue the APD at the dose effective for the acute phase? How long is treatment continued when symptoms have remitted? How long is an adequate treatment trial? And finally, can treatment ever be stopped? A trial of at least 8 weeks in adequate doses is needed to determine whether an antipsychotic is effective or not. In first episode patients response rates may cumulatively increase for up to 4 months (Gallego et al., 2011). However, there is also evidence that those patients showing a lack of response in the first 2 weeks may be non-responders in the longer run (Samara et al., 2015).

It is important to recognize that psychotic disorders are heterogeneous, and there is considerable variability in outcome with and without treatment. A small proportion of patients show remission after the first episode of psychosis, and may not require long-term medications (Harrow, Jobe, & Faull, 2012; Wunderink, et al., 2013). In most cases, however, treatment may need to be continued for life. After remission of an acute episode the same antipsychotic and the dose that was effective should be maintained for at least a year and probably longer. Discontinuing treatment at any point increases the risk of relapse. At this time, we have no way of predicting which patients need long-term treatment, and which ones may do well without medication.

Ensuring Compliance

Non-compliance, or a better term, non-adherence, is highly common in schizophrenia and related psychotic disorders, and can result from many factors, which may be patient-related (denial, lack of knowledge), illness-related (cognitive impairment, lack of insight, psychosis), or treatment-related (lack of efficacy, side effects, cost and impracticality of taking medications). Early identification of non-adherence is important, and management depends on the particular causes (Perkins, 2002). Long-acting, depot medications can be very helpful, and should be considered early in treatment in patients who tend to relapse because of non-adherence (Karson, 2016). Long-acting injectable (LAI) antipsychotics are highly recommended for non-adherent patients, though they can be useful in a broad range of patients and are worth considering early in treatment. Non-adherence is easier to detect with LAI, as it is evident as soon as a dose is missed. From the patients' point of view, LAIs remove the hassle of remembering to take a medication dose, and from the families' point of view, LAIs remove medication as a source of contentious struggles, especially in situations where the patient is reluctant to accept treatment.

Addressing Comorbidity

Comorbid medical illnesses, substance abuse, and depression are highly prevalent in schizophrenia, and can lead to setbacks in treatment response and functional recovery. Medical and substance abuse problems may have causal roles underlying psychotic symptoms and cognitive impairments (e.g. seizure disorders, head injury), and may be a consequence of disease or treatment effects (e.g. metabolic syndrome and weight gain). Comorbid disorders may also be simply coincidental but deserve attention because medical and substance use disorders are frequently missed in people with serious mental illnesses either because of the patients not seeking care or because of poor integration between mental health, medical and substance use services. Depressive symptoms are common over the course of schizophrenia (Koreen et al., 1993), and often resolve with antipsychotic monotherapy. However, if they are persistent and/or severe, a course of adjunctive antidepressant treatment may be worth considering.

Cannabis consumption and potency have seen a dramatic increase in the US in recent years. It is often difficult, but important to distinguish substance-induced psychosis from schizophrenia with substance use, since the former may not require long-term treatment with antipsychotics. Regular and heavy cannabis use can cause come cognitive impairment, although this issue remains debatable (Gonzalez et al., 2017); the clinician therefore needs to pay attention to addressing the comorbid substance use problem while embarking upon cognitive enhancement interventions.

Continuity of Care

An important, often underappreciated reason for relapses and poor outcome is the frequent change in care providers and care settings, which results from the fragmentation of care in public mental health settings and health care systems. We have seen patients relapse when their doctors change each time a resident or another trainee clinician shifts out at the end of a clinic rotation; it is therefore critical that the treatment team maintain continuity of at least some of its team members, plan for transitions and be alert to the effects of clinician change and take appropriate measures. Maintenance of therapeutic engagement enables an optimum long-term outcome. Discontinuities in care, either due to patients' relocation, or change in insurance, can increase risk of relapse or suboptimal treatment response, where possible, fragmentation of care should be avoided, and if inevitable, appropriate transition and overlap in care should be arranged.

Managing Side Effects

All antipsychotics have side effects, though some newer medications have a relatively better side effect profile (Table 7.1). Prevention is the best strategy, by appropriate choice of medication at the beginning, education, and early detection. When side effects emerge, dose reduction is a good first step; change to an alternative antipsychotic may then be considered. Problems with weight gain and metabolic side effects are best managed by healthy lifestyle programs, apart from the above measures. Problems with drug-induced Parkinsonism may be addressed with anticholinergic drugs, though their cognitive side effects are a limitation, as discussed later. Akathisia (restlessness) may require addition of a beta-blocker, a benzodiazepine or an antihistamine. Excessive sedation may be an initial problem until tolerance develops to the medication, but may warrant change in medication in some cases.

Managing Treatment Resistance

As noted, about a third of patients fail to respond after adequate trials of two or more antipsychotics. Persistent symptoms despite treatment should lead to consideration of (a) whether the trials were of adequate dose or duration; (b) covert non-adherence; (c) emergent medical illness; and (d) the possibility of diagnostic error. Clozapine should be considered in addressing treatment resistance, but has significant side effects, and needs to be carefully monitored.

Pharmacological "Subtraction"

The unfortunate tendency in clinical practice is for physicians to keep adding medications whenever treatment response is unsatisfactory. However, less is often more when it comes to psychotropic medications; pharmacological "subtraction" may often be more beneficial. Several psychotherapeutic drugs have negative effects on cognition. The case of Mary (see case study) illustrates this point. While the inpatient physicians' approach to add medications to her psychosis was well-intended, the combination of two antipsychotics, a tricyclic antidepressant, an antiparkinsonian drug (benztropine) and lithium created a large anticholinergic load. Anticholinergic agents which are commonly used to treat extrapyramidal side-effects of antipsychotics, frequently have cognitive side effects. Excessive and prolonged use of these agents can increase the likelihood of cognitive impairments in schizophrenia and other neuropsychiatric disorders. In Mary's case, the anticholinergic drugs led to her memory impairment, and the use of the benzodiazepine clonazepam added to her sedation.

Case Study 7.1

Mary is a 28-year-old unemployed woman with a diagnosis of schizophrenia which began when she was 22. She is currently single, unemployed, receives SSDI support and lives with her three young children, all below 5 years of age. She has been regularly attending the partial hospital program for the past 2 months. She had been stable till about 3 months ago when she had been briefly hospitalized for a psychotic relapse following a break up with her boyfriend. Her previous medications that she had been very compliant with i.e. clozapine 300 mg twice a day, amitriptyline 75 mg at night, and lithium carbonate 300 mg three times a day were continued. Perphenazine 32 mg at night, benztropine 1 mg twice a day, and clonazepam 1 mg twice a day had been added during the hospitalization.

One day, Mary did not show up for her partial hospital program and also did not come for her regular medical appointment that day. Since this was unusual for Mary, her case manager called and had no response. By the afternoon neighbors were concerned because children were crying loudly inside the house and Mary was not answering the door. The police were called and they entered the house to find Mary in a deep sleep. When she woke up, she admitted to having been very groggy and said she may have taken the morning medicines again because she "forgot."

Many antipsychotics also have anticholinergic effects. It is possible to assay the *in vivo* anticholinergicity of psychotropic drugs (in particular antipsychotics and tricyclic antidepressants) in serum and then examine its relation to cognition. There is evidence that serum anticholinergicity is correlated with cognitive dysfunction in schizophrenia, and that this relationship may be mediated by reductions in gray matter density (Wojtalik et al., 2012). This effect is dose-related. For these reasons, it is important to minimize the tendency to use many drugs (polypharmacy), and to use minimum effective doses, whenever possible, and if possible avoid psychotropic drugs with high anticholinergic effects such as chlorpromazine, thioridazine, and tricyclic antidepressants. Where necessary, switching to an appropriate atypical antipsychotic agent can help reduce the need for an anticholinergic agent.

7.2 Pro-cognitive Pharmacological Agents

Several studies including meta-analyses have shown that atypical antipsychotics may produce some cognitive improvement in people with schizophrenia compared to first generation antipsychotics (Keefe et al., 1999; Woodward et al., 2005). However, more recent analyses of data from the Clinical Antipsychotic Trials of Intervention Effectiveness (CATIE) and the European First Episode Schizophrenia Trial (EUFEST) studies failed to find differences between typical and atypical antipsychotics (Keefe, 2007). Many of these studies have been criticized on methodological grounds including the fact that most did not include control groups. This is important because it is possible that at least some of the improvements could be related to practice effects, given the fact that these studies include multiple repeated cognitive testing. In fact, the magnitude of the practice effects may be larger than the effects of the various medications (Goldberg et al., 2010). While sobering in regard to the potential beneficial effect of medications, this observation is a reminder of the powerful effect of repeated training on cognition, and a powerful rationale for psychosocial approaches to cognitive enhancement. Further, potential pharmacological targets to improve cognition, other than dopamine blockers, need to be investigated.

Several neurotransmitter systems are implicated in cognitive impairment in schizophrenia, suggesting that pharmacological options may have therapeutic benefits. Having a pharmacological agent that could improve cognition may have practical benefits since they can be administered on a daily basis without office visits and can provide continuous cognitive enhancement; they may also be cost-effective in the long run. A large number of studies have now been carried out to examine therapeutic benefits of a variety of pharmacological agents but the results thus far have been modest or disappointing. Figure 7.2 shows a list of these compounds organized by their mechanism of action.

Two classes of medications have shown some promise. First, amphetamine is one of the earliest drugs to be investigated for efficacy in the treatment of cognitive impairments in schizophrenia. One study (Barch & Carter, 2005) showed that single dose challenges with amphetamine resulted in enhancement of cognition across several domains. While promising, the long-term safety of stimulants for treating people with schizophrenia and risk of psychosis exacerbation might limit their use in this illness. Second, modafinil (a wakefulness-promoting medication used in narcolepsy) has shown some encouraging results. Early studies in patients with schizophrenia showed that modafinil improved cognitive flexibility, as indexed by the intra-extradimensional attentional set shifting task (Turner et al., 2004), in motor function (Farrow et al., 2006) and in clinical measures such as quality of life (Rosenthal & Braant, 2003). Modafinil has also been found to improve

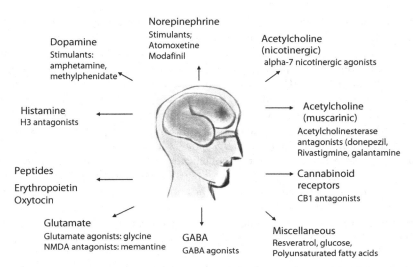

Figure 7.2 Several pharmacologic agents being tried now for cognitive deficits in schizophrenia, but have little or modest benefit. GABA = γ aminobutyric acid; NMDA = N-methyl D-aspartate. CB1= cannabinoid 1

cognition in patients with first episode psychoses (Scoriels et al., 2012). Modafinil has been shown in an fMRI study to increase dorsolateral prefrontal activity in schizophrenia patients with severe cognitive dysfunction (Hunter, 2006). However, a more recent double-blind controlled trial showed no differential effect on cognitive improvement when used adjunctively with cognitive training for 6 weeks (Michalopoulou et al., 2015).

Other neuroprotective agents have been investigated for potential pro-cognitive benefit. Notably, glucose administration has been demonstrated to improve cognition (particularly memory performance) in schizophrenia (reviewed in [Stone et al., 2003]). While regular glucose administration itself is an unlikely cognitive treatment due to negative metabolic side effects, it suggests the importance of glycemic status in cognition and the potential utility of novel types of pharmacological interventions. Erythropoietin (EPO), a drug which enhances synthesis of red blood cells, has been shown to have neuroprotective effects in animal models. There is some evidence from clinical trials that EPO is superior to placebo in treatment of cognitive deficits in schizophrenia (Ehrenreich et al., 2004). Potential adverse effects of EPO therapy may include increased risk of thrombosis, cancer, and hypertension. Resveratrol, a neuroprotective agent, has been tested for pro-cognitive effects in schizophrenia with negative results (Zortea et al., 2016). There is some evidence that cognitive impairment in schizophrenia may be associated with reductions in polyunsaturated fatty acids (Knöchel et al., 2015). However, there is no evidence that omega3 fatty acids have therapeutic benefits on cognition in this illness (Satogami et al., 2017). Intranasal oxytocin, a neuropeptide with known effects on social bonding, has been investigated for its potential benefits in improving social cognition in psychiatric disorders. A small, but significant effect was seen in a recent meta-analysis of 466 patients with a variety of neurodevelopmental disorders, including schizophrenia and autism spectrum disorders (Keech, Crowe, & Hocking, 2018). This effect was not moderated by the age, diagnosis or oxytocin dose. While promising, these observations must be considered tentative.

Several other drugs have been investigated, with little evidence of benefit. A controlled trial of MK-0777, a γ-aminobutyric acid (GABA)(A) α2/α3 partial agonist did not support initial promise of efficacy (Buchanan et al., 2011). Likewise, a controlled study of a H3 receptor antagonist GSK239512 did not show cognitive benefits in schizophrenia (Jarskog et al., 2015). Acetylcholinesterase inhibitors, such as donepezil and rivastigmine, have shown only modest, if any effects in schizophrenia (Singh, Kour, & Jayaram, 2012). Galantamine, a cholinesterase inhibitor, which also has effects on nicotinic acetylcholine receptors, has not shown efficacy for cognitive functions in schizophrenia (Lindenmayer & Khan, 2011). Alpha7 nicotinic acetylcholine receptor (α7 nAChR) agonists have not shown consistent efficacy for negative symptoms and cognitive impairment in schizophrenia (Deutsch et al., 2013). Memantine, an NMDA glutamate receptor antagonist drug used in dementia, has not shown benefit for cognitive deficits in schizophrenia in a double-blind controlled trial (Lieberman et al., 2009). In recent years the endocannabinoid system has also been investigated as a potential target for the treatment of schizophrenia. Two approaches have been used: antagonism of the cannabinoid 1 (CB1) receptors using drugs such as rimonabant and modulators of the endogenous cannabinoids such as cannabidiol. While some initial promising results have been found, thus far there has been no evidence for pro-cognitive effects of these compounds (Osborne, Solowij, & Weston-Green, 2017).

In summary, the literature of therapeutic use of pharmacological agents for cognitive deficits in schizophrenia remains mixed. Lack of effect of cognitive-enhancing drugs may be related to inadequate statistical power. Crossover designs can enhance power via within-subject analyses but may be limited by practice effects. It is also possible that improvements in neurocognitive deficits may be related to sample heterogeneity (e.g. genetic differences) but these may be addressed by future studies that use a stratified approach (Keshavan et al., 2017). One of the main reasons for the failure of many promising drugs in Phase 2 and Phase 3 studies is the high rate of placebo response. Several reasons may account for this: the pressure to enroll subjects with ambitious timelines and the financial incentives may encourage a tendency on quantity rather than quality and relax entry criteria leading to weaker results. Use of multiple sites for data collection may also lead to a dilution of quality. Another reason might be the use of well-known but insensitive measures of change in cognition and other outcome parameters. Use of smaller but higher quality sites, external verification of study entry criteria as well as centralized raters and objective laboratory-based measures of outcome assessment can potentially help in future studies (also see Chapter 11).

In contrast to patient populations, healthy people are increasingly using stimulants, such as amphetamine, methylphenidate, and modafinil, to enhance cognitive function. These "smart drugs" raise ethical as well as safety issues.

7.3 Neuromodulation and Cognitive Enhancement

Neuromodulation approaches such as Transcranial magnetic stimulation (TMS) are being used to modulate brain processes to address impairments in cognition (Lett et al., 2014). TMS uses a magnetic field generator, or "coil" connected to a pulse generator to produce small electric currents via electromagnetic induction just under the coil (see Figure 7.3). There are two types of TMS: single pulse, and repetitive; effects are longer

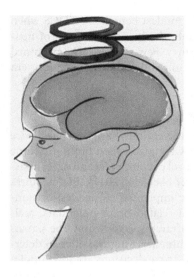

Figure 7.3 Transcranial magnetic stimulation using a figure 8 coil

lasting with the latter (rTMS). Neuronal activity is increased in rTMS when a higher frequency (e.g. 5–10 HZ) is used and decreased when a lower frequency (i.e. 1 HZ) is used. rTMS modulates local inhibitory circuits thereby facilitating or inhibiting neural circuits. Several studies suggest that rTMS applied to the dorsolateral prefrontal cortex (DLPFC) can variably impair encoding and retrieval of visuospatial and verbal stimuli (Rossi et al., 2001) or facilitate cognitive processes such as object naming and psychomotor speed (Boroojerdi et al., 2001; Cappa et al., 2002). The relation between regional brain function and cognitive performance can be examined, by investigating how TMS-induced changes in DLPFC activity relate to cognitive function. Combining TMS with EEG (TMS-EEG) allows measurement of both temporal and spatial activations at the targeted brain regions (Rogasch & Fitzgerald, 2013).

Over the past decade, a large literature has emerged on the potential effects of rTMS in enhancing cognition. The mechanisms remain unclear. First, it is possible that the rTMS directly modulates neural circuitries underlying impaired cognition. Cognitive impairments in psychiatric disorders such as schizophrenia have been thought to be related to abnormalities in neural oscillations such as gamma synchrony (Spencer et al., 2004). Such alterations have in turn been attributed to impaired functioning of GABA interneurons and cortico–cortical interactions (Lewis, 2014). Second, there is increasing evidence that cognitive impairments may result from impairments in brain plasticity (see Chapter 1). It is possible that rTMS enhances brain plasticity, and thereby facilitates Hebbian learning. Limited evidence suggests the potential benefit of rTMS in improving cognition across several neuropsychiatric disorders (Demirtas-Tatlidede, Vahabzadeh-Hagh, & Pascual-Leone, 2013), though one controlled study showed negative results (Rabany, Deutsch, & Levkovitz, 2014).

Another approach to neuromodulation is transcranial direct current stimulation (TDCS), which uses-low grade constant electrical stimulation to brain regions using a simple device. It has some uses in depression; a few studies have evaluated its value in treating cognitive deficits and a recent review suggests modest benefits of TDCS when applied to the left DLPFC (Mervis et al., 2017). Overall, the beneficial effects of neuromodulation on cognition is a promising line of inquiry. Few studies have examined whether simultaneous administration of neuromodulation and cognitive enhancement techniques can have synergistic effects.

Brain–Computer Interfaces and Neurofeedback

Neuromodulation as discussed above is a one-way intervention – an external device changing brain function. Brain–computer interface (BCIs), also called brain–machine interface, approaches involve the opposite: enabling control of computers and other assistive devices by using signals from the brain (Lebedev & Nicolelis, 2017). BCI acquires signals of interest either directly from the brain, using implanted electrodes, or non-invasively using electroencephalographic signals, event-related brain potentials, real-time functional magnetic resonance imaging, or near-infrared spectroscopy. The signals will then have to be extracted and processed via a machine learning classifier to determine mental states (e.g. intent to press a button or not). These decisions are then implemented via control signals to an external device, such as a computer cursor, a monitor to provide visual and/or auditory feedback, a robotic arm or even to stimulate the brain via neuromodulation. The addition of neurofeedback in BCI makes the interventional approach bidirectional (Figure 7.4).

BCIs offer an alternative way of responding to the world, when normal output pathways such as nerves and muscles are not functioning. A classic example is "locked in" syndrome, a neurological condition in which the affected person is awake, but unable to move or communicate because of total motor paralysis. Patients with other neurological conditions such as aphasias may also benefit from BCIs. Patients with severe dementia, who are unable to communicate verbally, could benefit from a BCI to respond with basic

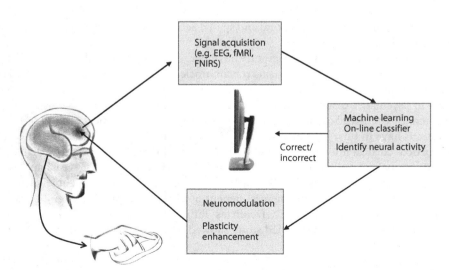

Figure 7.4 Brain computer interface: a schematic diagram. EEG: Electroencephalogram. fMRI: Functional Magnetic Resonance Imaging. FNIRS: Functional Near-Infrared Spectroscopy

(e.g. "yes" and "no") to cognitively demanding tasks. Though BCI and neurofeedback studies are beginning to appear in psychiatric disorders such as autism spectrum disorders, very few studies have been published using BCIs for cognitive enhancement in schizophrenia (Carelli et al., 2017).

Making things happen just by thinking about them is no longer in the realm of science fiction alone. However, progress has been slow, because of several road-blocks which limit application of BCIs: lack of reliable neural patterns that distinguish mental states; limited speed (e.g. commands per minute), need for extensive training to use BCI, and user fatigue. The loss of autonomy may also be a concern. The question of who gets enhanced memory when such technology becomes available also raises ethical problems of social justice.

7.4 Summary

- Stabilization of symptoms by optimal use of antipsychotics and other psychotropic medication is a critical prerequisite for the success of cognitive enhancement interventions.
- Optimum pharmacotherapy requires comprehensive assessment, an integrated care plan, and careful attention to therapeutic alliance, appropriate choice of the medication(s), adherence, comorbidity, and side effect issues.
- Cognitive benefits can be gained by avoiding unnecessary and excessive use of medications, and also minimizing the use of drugs that can have negative cognitive effects, such as anticholinergics.
- Several medications have been tested for possible efficacy in improving cognition in schizophrenia and related disorders, but so far with little or modest benefit. Neuromodulation techniques such as TMS may have a potential for cognitive enhancement.
- Brain–computer interface and neurofeedback approaches as a way to enhance cognition is at an early developmental phase, and more research is needed.

Personalizing and Optimizing Cognitive Enhancement

8

Who Responds Best? Predictors and Moderators of Cognitive Enhancement

8.1 Introduction

Cognitive enhancement is the systematic practice of cognitive exercises, strategic training, and approaches to compensate for cognitive challenges to address the social and non-social cognitive factors that limit functional recovery from schizophrenia and related conditions. Meta-analytic evidence has consistently indicated a benefit of cognitive enhancement approaches on diverse cognitive outcomes, symptomatology, and functioning in patients with schizophrenia (McGurk et al., 2007; Wykes et al., 2011), leading to its establishment as an evidence-based practice and one of the only effective approaches for addressing core cognitive impairments in this population. While such evidence has indeed ushered in a new generation of treatment options for patients (Eack, 2012), it is important to remember that effect sizes and outcome results are based on analyses of groups of patients, not individuals.

Schizophrenia is a remarkably heterogeneous condition, so much so that some believe that several distinct disorders are currently included in this category (Clementz et al., 2016). Some patients with schizophrenia have a rapid onset characterized predominantly by positive symptoms and respond well to antipsychotic medication. Others have a more gradual onset with greater degree of negative symptoms that do not respond as well to first-line antipsychotic treatments. Prognosis is highly variable, as is symptom response to pharmacotherapy. Some individuals are able to recover more quickly, return to school or work, and live meaningful and satisfying lives, whereas other individuals struggle for years trying to come to terms with their condition and gain some level of symptomatic and functional recovery. Although there are few guarantees when working with patients with schizophrenia, heterogeneity is one of the few characteristics that a clinician can count on and expect to see throughout her practice with this population.

Cognition and cognitive impairments are no exception to the heterogeneity so frequently observed among patients with schizophrenia. Some patients may experience significant problems in memory, particularly working memory for verbal instructions, conversations, and other spoken language. Others may have challenges in processing speed and attention, and have great difficulty in completing tasks quickly and attending to important information in the environment. Still other patients will experience difficulties in planning ahead and solving everyday problems, sometimes referred to as executive function or problem-solving (see Chapter 1). To see one person with schizophrenia and to come to know his cognitive difficulties leaves little guarantee of the cognitive presentation of the next person encountered with the condition. In one of the most comprehensive reviews of neurocognitive impairment in schizophrenia, Heinrichs and Zakzanis (1998) examined performance of nearly 2 dozen cognitive abilities and tests in patients with the condition compared to healthy volunteers. Ranking domains from the most to the least impaired, on average, they found that schizophrenia was associated with large impairments in verbal memory ($d = 1.41$), motor skill ($d = 1.30$), attention ($d = 1.16$), verbal fluency ($d = 1.15$), and cognitive flexibility ($d = 1.11$). The least impaired were the domains of basic working memory for numbers ($d = 0.61$), line orientation judgments ($d = 0.60$), basic vocabulary ($d = 0.53$), and visual–spatial problem-solving ($d = 0.46$). With even the largest domain of impairment, however, some 20% of patients still perform within normal ranges, and as many as 60% of patients evidence significant impairments even on cognitive domains least impaired in the disorder (Heinrichs & Zakzanis, 1998). Clearly the neurocognitive presentation of individuals living with schizophrenia is highly heterogeneous.

Social-cognitive impairments follow a similar and perhaps even more heterogeneous pattern. While domains of social cognition are still being investigated and assessments currently are not as established as those associated with neurocognitive function, most consider social cognition to include theory of mind, social perception, attributional biases, emotion perception, and emotion processing (see Chapter 1 for more details). A comprehensive meta-analytic review by Savla et al. (2012) found social perception ($d = 1.04$) and theory of mind ($d = 0.96$) to be the two largest social-cognitive domains of impairment in schizophrenia, whereas attributional biases, both personalizing ($d = -0.17$) and externalizing ($d = -0.02$), were least impaired. However, results again evidenced considerable heterogeneity, with 95% of effect sizes for theory of mind ranging between large ($d = 0.83$) and very large ($d = 1.09$) impairments. Clearly people with schizophrenia have significant impairments in theory of mind, but on average, these impairments vary widely and not all individuals may evidence an impairment that is clinically significant. Conversely, 95% of effect sizes for attributional biases ranged from higher functioning than healthy volunteers ($d = -0.72$) to small ($d = 0.37$) impairments, suggesting that some patients have deficits in attributional style, but that most do not exhibit such impairments. It seems that regardless of the cognitive construct under study, heterogeneity in presentation can be assumed and no single profile of cognitive impairments best describes patients with schizophrenia.

To address this issue and facilitate the treatment of heterogeneous cognitive challenges in patients with schizophrenia, Hogarty and colleagues (Hogarty et al., 2004) developed and applied a novel concept of cognitive styles to the treatment of cognitive impairment in this population. They formulated three styles of impaired cognition that are prominently represented across diverse patients with schizophrenia, and such styles became organizing heuristics in guiding the application of Cognitive Enhancement Therapy (CET) to people with the condition. The three cognitive styles were identified from reviews of the literature and the decades of experience this group had in the treatment of schizophrenia, and consisted of *unmotivated*, *disorganized*, and *inflexible* cognitive styles (see Table 8.1 and Chapter 3). Hogarty and colleagues viewed these cognitive styles as dimensional in nature and potentially overlapping, such that a patient may demonstrate aspects of more than one cognitive style. However, in most cases, a single cognitive style will be predominant and will be the focus of treatment in CET.

Table 8.1 Cognitive styles as an organizing principle for the heterogeneity of cognitive impairment in schizophrenia

Cognitive style	Functional characteristics
Unmotivated style	Challenges with motivation, low-energy level, difficulty using elaborated speech, reduced mental stamina, problems generating ideas, difficulty using active thinking
Disorganized style	Challenges with organizing concepts, excessive focus on details rather than the gist, difficulty using language coherently, emotional "flooding"
Inflexible style	Challenges with considering alternative perspectives and solutions to problems, fixed routines, stereotypic views of people and relationships, intolerance of ambiguity, excessive discomfort with new situations

Note: See Hogarty and Greenwald (2006) for greater discussion of cognitive styles and their application to treatment using CET.

The concept of cognitive styles has primarily been used as an organizing heuristic for parsing the heterogeneity of cognitive challenges patients present with for treatment, particularly in CET. This concept has served well in helping clinicians identify targets for cognitive enhancement interventions and linking those targets to functional behaviors, such as reduced mental stamina at school or challenges in organizing what to say in conversations. The empirical investigation of cognitive styles has received comparatively less attention. The original study of CET found that unmotivated and disorganized cognitive styles tended to be most common among patients with schizophrenia, and that multiple dominant cognitive styles were apparent in less than 10% of the sample. Perhaps not surprisingly, unmotivated and disorganized styles were most responsive to CET treatment, whereas patients with the inflexible style evidenced somewhat less improvement, but this was relatively less than those with the other two styles. Currently, whether cognitive style predicts specific treatment response to cognitive enhancement, beyond degree of improvement, is not known for CET or other rehabilitation interventions. What is clear, however, is that these styles characterize much of what a clinician will see when treating cognitive problems in schizophrenia and related disorders, and help to guide the treatment of this population by reducing the heterogeneity observed around three specific styles of information processing impairment.

While the concept of cognitive styles is useful for guiding cognitive enhancement interventions, and helps to address heterogeneity in initial presentation, variability continues to ensue in treatment response and outcomes from rehabilitation programs. The systematic investigation of moderators of cognitive enhancement is only beginning, and little empirical evidence is available to guide clinicians in the selection of appropriate patients. What follows is a presentation of the main moderating factors that have been observed in the treatment of cognitive impairment in schizophrenia. Because of the emerging state of this field, much of the information provided comes from our clinical experience in providing cognitive enhancement interventions, in addition to the small but growing body of literature in this area (see Table 8.2).

8.2 Symptom Stability

Positive symptom stability is a critical factor in many psychosocial treatments for schizophrenia. Although certainly not required for all interventions, early research has clearly indicated that the benefits of psychosocial treatment for this population will be greatest

Table 8.2 Moderators of response to cognitive enhancement for schizophrenia

Moderator	Description
Symptom stability	Cognitive enhancement interventions are designed primarily for symptomatically stable outpatients who have good control of their positive symptoms through antipsychotic and psychosocial treatment. Studies suggest that more symptomatic patients benefit less from cognitive training.
Intellectual functioning	Nearly all of the cognitive enhancement evidence in schizophrenia has been evaluated in patients with IQ scores of 80 or higher. There is unclear benefit for those individuals with comorbid intellectual disability.
Substance use	The majority of studies of cognitive enhancement in schizophrenia have excluded patients with co-occurring substance use disorders, a significant proportion of the schizophrenia population. Studies that include patients with substance use problems have found that cognitive enhancement can be efficacious in the presence of comorbid substance use disorder, but with higher rates of treatment discontinuation.
Course of illness	Cognitive enhancement is effective for long-term and early course schizophrenia patients. The use of cognitive enhancement as an early intervention strategy can significantly enhance effects on functional outcome and may capitalize on neuroplasticity reserves.
Psychosis diagnosis	Cognitive enhancement appears to be broadly effective for patients with schizophrenia, schizoaffective disorder, and schizophreniform disorder. There is no evidence of differential outcomes within the schizophrenia-spectrum, and there is emerging evidence of efficacy in bipolar disorder and other affective psychoses.
Biological markers	Cognitive cortical reserve, neurotrophic factors, and functional neural neuroimaging activity and connectivity (as measured by functional imaging) are emerging biological markers of response to cognitive remediation interventions. Evidence increasingly indicates that the neurobiological make-up of the patient prior to treatment is an important factor in predicting treatment response.

when patients experience some control and stability over their positive symptoms with antipsychotic treatment (Hogarty et al., 1974). When patients are acutely ill and experience increased positive symptoms that may require hospitalization, psychosocial interventions such as cognitive rehabilitation, supportive employment, and social skills training can prove to be overstimulating and may in fact exacerbate psychiatric symptoms. In most cases, intensive psychosocial treatment is best considered once appropriate, tolerable, and effective antipsychotic medication has been implemented (but see Chapters 4 and 7, along with Personal Therapy [Hogarty, 2002], Cognitive Behavioral Therapy for Psychosis [Kingdon & Turkington, 1994], and Assertive Community Treatment [Stein, 1980] as notable examples of psychosocial interventions that can help with symptom stabilization). Cognitive rehabilitation is no exception to this principle, and studies of cognitive enhancement interventions commonly have been restricted to stabilized patients with schizophrenia. Meta-analytic reviews of inpatient and outpatient studies of cognitive rehabilitation indicate that when symptom levels are higher, cognitive improvements associated with rehabilitation tend to be modest (Wykes et al., 2011). This is not surprising, as cognitive rehabilitation interventions have been conceptualized largely as stabilization-phase treatments that focus on improving functional recovery through the treatment of cognitive impairments (Eack, 2012). Although effects on symptoms have been observed in a number of studies (McGurk et al., 2007b), these symptom reductions are modest and do not necessarily indicate improvements in positive symptoms, but may reflect negative symptom improvement associated with cognitive gains (Eack, 2013).

It is important to recognize, however, that symptom stability does not mean the absence of positive or other psychiatric symptoms. Many patients with schizophrenia and related disorders experience ongoing challenges with positive symptoms, even with adequate antipsychotic treatment (Robinson et al., 2004). If the clinician were to wait for such symptoms to completely abate, few patients would be eligible for cognitive enhancement and many, while eligible, would have to wait years before beginning such treatment. It is important to begin treating the cognitive challenges associated with schizophrenia as soon as possible, so that the functional impairments to which these challenges contribute do not grow and patients are able to gain a greater functional recovery from their condition as soon as possible. As such, waiting for the perfect symptom presentation is not practical or helpful in the majority of cases who experience the condition. The clinician should seek primarily to determine that positive psychotic symptoms are below the threshold that would ordinarily result in hospitalization, such as when a patient is grossly disorganized and unable to speak coherently or when he is preoccupied and acting on hallucinatory or delusional symptoms. In such cases, group-based social cognition training is often not feasible or productive, and while computer-based training may be possible, patients with these symptoms have difficulty attending to rehabilitation tasks that makes them less effective, if beneficial at all.

With proper antipsychotic treatment, many patients with schizophrenia are able to achieve reduction in symptoms well below the threshold that would ordinarily result in hospitalization. The introduction of clozapine, in particular, allowed even more treatment-resistant patients a much better level of control over their psychotic symptoms (Siskind et al., 2016). Once the absolute threshold of positive psychotic symptoms has fallen below that which would be associated with a need for hospitalization, and appropriate time has been given to allow the patient to recover from an acute episode, the clinician can begin monitoring symptom stability to determine suitability for cognitive rehabilitation. Although the complete absence of positive symptoms is not required, a pattern of stability is essential for increasing the likelihood of a beneficial rehabilitation experience. Symptom levels that frequently change and increase to near-acute thresholds should be a cause of concern and met with hesitancy in starting rehabilitation. In contrast, positive symptoms that are present, only mildly interfering for the patient, and have shown a consistent or decreasing level for several prior months indicate a stability pattern favorable for beginning cognitive rehabilitation (see Figure 8.1).

8.3 Intellectual Functioning

Cognitive enhancement approaches are focused on improving cognitive performance in such domains as attention, working memory, and problem-solving in unrehearsed and novel situations. As studies of rehabilitation interventions have emerged for patients with schizophrenia and related conditions, the intellectual functioning of the patient has become recognized as an important predictor of treatment outcome. As pervasive and broad as cognitive impairments are in schizophrenia, cognitive rehabilitation remains focused on targeted deficits rather than generalized intellectual impairments. There is no evidence indicating that rehabilitation interventions are effective for improving overall IQ, treating comorbid intellectual disability in schizophrenia, or addressing the

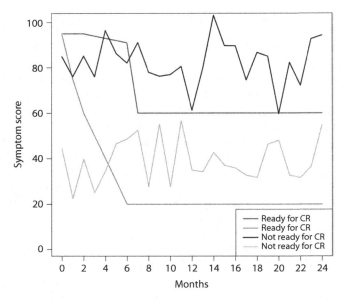

Figure 8.1 Patterns of symptom stability and readiness for cognitive rehabilitation

generalized impairments associated with low intellectual functioning. In fact, studies that examine the impact of cognitive rehabilitation among schizophrenia patients with lower intellectual functioning or comorbid intellectual disability have often found their approaches to be ineffective and less applicable to such individuals (e.g. Hogarty et al., 2004). As a consequence, the majority of clinical trials of cognitive training approaches in schizophrenia exclude individuals with IQ less than 70 or 80, due to the lack of benefit of these interventions for people with general intellectual impairments.

Of course, it must be recognized that many of the assessments employed that make up the cognitive rehabilitation evidence base in schizophrenia are derived directly or indirectly from intelligence tests. This can be confusing to clinicians, family members, and patients, as such findings would seem to suggest that cognitive enhancement can improve IQ. However, it is the fluid aspects of intelligence that are most commonly measured in rehabilitation studies, which serve as indexes of domain-specific performance in such areas as attention or problem-solving. More crystallized processes, such as language and vocabulary knowledge, are neither targeted nor appreciably changed with extant rehabilitation programs. As such, patients with generalized intellectual impairments find a relatively modest benefit from cognitive rehabilitation, and in most cases should receive alternative treatment more suited to their needs, such as Cognitive Adaptation Training (Velligan et al., 2000). Particularly challenging in people with lower intellectual ability is social cognition training, which often relies upon a more advanced vocabulary and conceptual understanding. For example, early trials of CET found that the social-cognitive group curriculum was difficult for patients with lower IQ to understand and that such patients improved less on a dozen different measures than individuals with higher IQ levels (Hogarty et al., 2004). Computer-based neurocognitive training may be more feasible with intellectually disabled patients, although the current literature has largely not evaluated the feasibility and impact of such interventions with this population. Cognitive enhancement interventions have recently been successfully adapted to populations with intellectual impairments such as velocardiofacial syndrome (Shashi et al., 2015) and autism (Eack et al., 2017), and been found to have therapeutic benefits. Clearly, more work is needed to scale up cognitive enhancement interventions to the broad spectrum of developmental disorders.

To be clear, many patients with schizophrenia have lower IQ scores within the 85–100 point range (Heinrichs & Zakzanis, 1998), as the information processing impairments individuals experience are detectable by many intelligence tests. Although such scores are lower, they remain within the normative range of overall intellectual functioning, and cognitive enhancement with such individuals is common, feasible, and often effective. As IQ moves closer to 80, practitioners are likely to find challenges in treatment, and especially when working with patients with an IQ less than 80. Cognitive enhancement can be adapted for this population, and there are many alternative intervention programs to support people with intellectual disability, such as token economy and other behaviorally oriented treatments (Szymanski & King, 1999).

8.4 Substance Use

Schizophrenia is known to co-occur with substance misuse and addiction challenges with a high degree of frequency, particularly nicotine, cannabis, and alcohol use (Volkow, 2009). Because such substances have significant impact on cognitive functioning, the majority of research trials of cognitive remediation interventions have excluded individuals who misuse alcohol and illicit substances. The concern has been that the negative cognitive impact of these drugs would interfere with the ability of patients to benefit from cognitive training programs, and therefore many recommend that those with substance use challenges first address those challenges before entering cognitive rehabilitation. Unfortunately, the prevalence of addiction issues in schizophrenia is so exceedingly high, and the response to addiction treatment relatively low, that such guidance could leave 30–50% of patients with schizophrenia ineligible for cognitive remediation. The concern about the cognitive impact of drugs of abuse is warranted, but largely untested, and there is emerging evidence that cognitive training approaches may also be useful for treating substance use problems (Wiers et al., 2013). Further, untested concerns about the impact of comorbid substance use on treatment response have to be balanced with the public health needs of society, where patients with schizophrenia and co-occurring substance use challenges are frequently encountered in everyday practice.

There are notable exceptions in research trials that have included schizophrenia patients with significant substance use problems, and the findings of these studies suggest that it may be both feasible and beneficial to include patients with schizophrenia and co-occurring addictions in cognitive enhancement programs. The work of McGurk and colleagues is particularly illustrative, as they have repeatedly conducted community-based effectiveness studies of cognitive training interventions combined with supported employment using samples of patients that very much reflect the "real world." For example, in their latest trial of Thinking Skills for Work, a cognitive training program combined with supported employment to improve work outcomes for those who did not respond to traditional supported employment interventions, 30% of included patients had a current substance use disorder and 60% of patients had a lifetime history of substance use problems. Patients receiving the Thinking Skills for Work Treatment engaged in competitive employment for over 3 months longer than traditional supported employment, earned twice as much money, and were employed in competitive jobs at nearly twice the rate of those not receiving the cognitive training intervention (McGurk et al., 2015). Clearly, these results show that cognitive training with patients with co-occurring addiction challenges is feasible and that significant benefits to meaningful functional outcomes can be obtained in this population. Such findings are largely consistent with their previous trials that included patients with substance use disorder (McGurk, 2005; McGurk et al., 2007a).

A recent, small pilot study by our own group using CET specifically sought to examine the feasibility of including patients with moderate cannabis or alcohol use problem, two of the most common drugs of abuse in schizophrenia. Unlike most other cognitive remediation trials, to enter the study patients had to have a diagnosis of schizophrenia or schizoaffective disorder, and meet criteria for moderate or greater cannabis or alcohol use problems. Results indicated large and significant improvements in neurocognition, social cognition, and social adjustment (Eack et al., 2015) at levels that were similar to previous trials in non-substance using patients (Eack et al., 2009; Hogarty et al., 2004). Further, more patients receiving CET reduced their alcohol, but not cannabis, use than those receiving the usual care condition, suggesting that cognitive remediation may help improve some substance use outcomes in this population (Eack et al., 2016). What was very different in this trial was not a reduced level of efficacy of CET, but a significantly greater attrition rate than we had observed in previous trials. Only 53% of substance misusing schizophrenia patients randomized to CET completed the full 18-month treatment, a marked reduction in treatment retention compared to non-substance using samples that routinely show 75% or greater retention over the course of CET (Eack et al., 2009; Hogarty et al., 2004). While certainly preliminary, these findings combined with those of McGurk and colleagues increasingly suggest that cognitive remediation can be extended to patients with schizophrenia who have co-occurring substance use disorder. Like most other studies of patients with addiction challenges, however, a higher dropout rate can be expected (Dutra et al., 2008).

Finally, it is important to note that our studies and those by other groups who include patients with schizophrenia and co-occurring substance use disorder frequently do not include those with the most severe addiction challenges, such as patients with opiate or cocaine dependence. In many cases, the addiction challenges were limited to alcohol and cannabis, and while significant, these challenges did not rise to the severity of substance use problems seen with opiates and other highly addictive illicit substances. While we advocate for the inclusion of all patients who can benefit in cognitive remediation, we also believe that those with the most severe addiction challenges would benefit from substance use treatment prior to beginning cognitive remediation.

8.5 Early versus Chronic Phase of Illness

The past two decades have seen a surge of interest in early intervention programs for patients with schizophrenia, as reflected by the National Institute of Mental Health "Recovery After an Initial Schizophrenia Episode" trial (National Institute of Mental Health, 2012) and an explosion of studies focused on early intervention and prevention of disability in schizophrenia (Marshall & Rathbone, 2011). It is widely documented that the longer the duration between the onset of psychosis and treatment, the poorer the prognosis (Perkins et al., 2005). Such evidence has highlighted the importance of intervening early in the course of psychotic disorders to prevent disability and help individuals make as rapid an adjustment to their condition as possible. Cognitive enhancement studies have now been conducted across a range of phases of illness, from the earliest phases of the onset of schizophrenia to those who have been living with the chronic condition for decades.

Initial studies of cognitive enhancement interventions were conducted in samples of patients with schizophrenia who had been ill for a decade or more. Findings from such studies largely indicated the benefits of cognitive remediation programs for enhancing neurocognitive abilities in processing speed, attention, verbal memory, and executive functioning (McGurk et al., 2007b). Some unique programs also demonstrated considerable benefits to social cognition, medication management, and psychiatric symptoms (Hogarty et al., 2004; Velligan et al., 2000). In fact, the majority of the evidence base supporting cognitive rehabilitation for the treatment of schizophrenia has been built on studies of patients with long-term, chronic schizophrenia. Consequently, we know the most about treating people with schizophrenia who have been through the initial (or several) acute episodes, have been stabilized on antipsychotic treatment, and are within in the later, recovery-phase of the condition. In many respects, this is the ideal target population for cognitive remediation interventions that seek to help patients move to the next chapter in their recovery. Those who have been ill for a number of years have had time to adjust to the condition, accept its presence and limitations, identify a tolerable and effective medication regimen, and look for tools to further their recovery beyond medication management. As such, long-term patients with schizophrenia can be an ideal population for whom to implement cognitive enhancement interventions, and given the evidence base, the practitioner can be optimistic about the potential for such treatments to produce meaningful improvements in people who have been living with the condition for many years.

At the same time, the early phase of schizophrenia offers an unparalleled therapeutic window for intervention and prevention of later disability. Cognitive impairments associated with schizophrenia begin early (Mesholam-Gately et al., 2009), perhaps even before the onset of frank psychotic symptoms (Bora & Murray, 2013), and they are largely unresponsive to antipsychotic medications (Keefe et al., 2007). Further, some have hypothesized that in the first several years of illness onset, the brain retains neuroplastic reserves that make it uniquely capable of benefiting from cognitive remediation (Keshavan, 1999), and thus the power of cognitive training may be significantly enhanced by intervening early in the course of the disorder. While evidence regarding this hypothesis is still emerging (Bowie et al., 2013; Revell et al., 2015), what is clearly known is that functional recovery from schizophrenia becomes more and more difficult the longer a person is disabled. Registration for disability supports is a very concrete example of this phenomenon. Many young people with schizophrenia have recently been involved in work or school, and often receive their health insurance coverage in the US through their parents or caregivers. Conversely, older individuals who have been living with schizophrenia for 5 or more years often find that they need to register for disability supports, including Social Security Disability benefits and Medicaid for health insurance coverage. As the years since last employment or schooling increases, individuals find it increasingly difficult to re-enter the work or school system. Further, as reliance on the disability system lengthens, many individuals find it difficult to obtain competitive employment that would provide sufficient financial and health insurance coverage. Many long-term patients find themselves in the disability trap, where they want to work and contribute, but do not want to jeopardize their financial or medical security, and the jobs available are not high-paying enough to cover their medical needs. These issues become worse the longer a person has a disability, presenting structural barriers to functional recovery, and therefore the earlier one can intervene, the more likely the patient will be able to get back on track with work or school and not become entrenched in the disability system.

Studies of cognitive enhancement interventions for patients in the early course of schizophrenia are only recently emerging, and certainly too few exist at this time to determine whether there is a marked difference in response to treatment between those in the early versus chronic phases of the condition. Extant evidence does suggest, however, that the benefits may be considerable. In one of the few head-to-head comparisons, Bowie and colleagues treated patients in the early course (5 years or less) or chronic phase (15 years or longer) of schizophrenia with 12 weeks of neurocognitive training, and found improvements in cognition and functional outcomes, particularly work skills, to be significantly greater in the early course sample (Bowie et al., 2013). In studies of CET, patients in the early course of schizophrenia showed less improvement in processing speed than those who had been ill for longer periods of time, possibly because of the more intact processing speed scores at the earlier phases of the condition (Eack et al., 2009). However, improvements in social cognition and functional outcome, particularly competitive employment, were markedly increased when treating patients in the early course of schizophrenia. Such effects are illustrative of the potential of early intervention with cognitive remediation to support meaningful functional gains in schizophrenia and related conditions, and while cognitive training interventions are clearly effective for those who have been ill for decades or more, the sooner cognitive remediation interventions can be applied the greater the opportunity for functional recovery and prevention of disability.

8.6 Schizophrenia versus Other Psychoses

The treatment of cognitive challenges using cognitive enhancement approaches in schizophrenia has largely been evaluated in samples of patients with *schizophrenia-spectrum disorders*, which have included primarily individuals diagnosed with schizophrenia, schizoaffective disorder, or schizophreniform disorder. Few studies in the literature make the distinction between schizophrenia and schizoaffective disorder, a form of schizophrenia that also includes significant mood dysfunction, such as depression or mania (American Psychiatric Association, 2013). As such, the efficacy of cognitive enhancement interventions is broadly thought to extend not only to patients with schizophrenia, but also to those individuals with schizoaffective disorder and schizophreniform disorder (particularly those cases that continue to experience symptoms, and that ultimately develop into schizophrenia). A meta-analytic review of studies of cognitive enhancement with patients with schizoaffective disorder, bipolar disorder, and other affective psychoses found somewhat reduced, but largely similar effect sizes for improving cognition as found in studies of patients with schizophrenia (Anaya et al., 2012). A comparison of early course patients with schizophrenia or schizoaffective disorder treated with CET found equivalent levels of cognitive improvement between the two conditions (Lewandowski et al., 2011), further indicating that the benefits of cognitive remediation can be extended to those with schizoaffective disorder. Finally, non-schizophrenia psychotic disorders may also benefit from cognitive enhancement interventions. Lewandowski and colleagues (Lewandowski, Ongur, & Keshavan, 2017) showed benefits of a computer-based cognitive remediation program with bridging groups compared to an active intervention in psychotic bipolar patients.

The findings that cognitive enhancement appears to be similarly effective for patients with schizophrenia and affective psychoses are aligned with emerging evidence for an overlapping biological substratum for these two conditions (Mathew et al., 2014). In fact, with the National Institute of Mental Health Research Domains of Criteria (RDoC) initiative (Insel et al., 2010), many questions are being raised about traditional psychiatric nosology and its alignment, or lack thereof, with biological markers for disorder. While affective psychoses clearly present additional mood-related challenges not evident in schizophrenia, research on the underlying neural mechanisms contributing to cognitive impairment across the psychosis spectrum suggests common abnormalities that may transcend individual psychotic conditions (Clementz et al., 2016). The practitioner, therefore, should consider the inclusion of patients with schizoaffective disorder in their cognitive enhancement programs, as these interventions appear to have benefits across the schizophrenia spectrum.

8.7 Emerging Biomoderators

Clinical factors have had a major role in research on predictors and moderators of response to cognitive enhancement interventions. Symptom stability, substance use comorbidity, cognitive style, phase of illness, and intellectual disability all have a significant moderating impact on response to cognitive remediation. In recent years, the field has expanded its investigation of moderators of cognitive training outcomes well beyond behavioral clinical variables and has begun to examine biological markers that may predict treatment response, what we refer to as *biomoderators*. Some of the earliest work in this area has been conducted with magnetic resonance imaging and predicting cognitive training outcomes from pre-treatment neurobiological characteristics. For example, Keshavan and colleagues found that patients with greater pre-treatment cortical gray matter demonstrated a more rapid social-cognitive response to CET compared to those patients with less cortical gray matter (Keshavan et al., 2011). This led Keshavan and colleagues to hypothesize that greater structural neurobiological reserves may portend a particularly rapid response to cognitive remediation and enable patients to obtain the same benefit from the treatment with shorter exposure. The concept of a cortical reserve originated from the Alzheimer's disease literature, and suggests that some neurobiological redundancy or compensatory mechanisms may exist that protect against illness manifestation (Stern, 2012). In the case of cognitive enhancement in schizophrenia, such reserves may be associated with a greater capacity for neuroplasticity that could contribute to an accelerated treatment response.

Neurotrophic factors are proteins that regulate neuron proliferation and migration, and many of them, such as brain-derived neurotrophic factor, are thought to be markers of neuroplasticity or neuroplastic capacity (Autry & Monteggia, 2012). Their role in neurodevelopment and neuroprotection makes neurotrophic factors likely candidates for markers and predictors of cognitive improvement during cognitive remediation. To date, many studies have documented decreases in serum brain-derived neurotrophic factor in schizophrenia, but few have examined the role of this factor in cognitive remediation. One study by Vinogradov and colleagues found that plasticity-based auditory training was associated with significant increases in brain-derived neurotrophic factor. Further, the increases in this factor were associated with significant improvements in quality of life, suggesting that they may have served as mechanisms for improved outcomes (Vinogradov et al., 2009). Another study found that schizophrenia patients with genetic abnormalities that reduced BDNF expression in the brain were less likely to benefit from cognitive enhancement (Bosia et al., 2014).

Finally, functional neuroimaging studies have been rapidly emerging indicating that various measures of brain function may index cognitive improvement during cognitive enhancement for schizophrenia. In a recent study of CET, investigators found that CET was associated with significant increases in dorsolateral prefrontal cortical activity, which were related to improvements in cognitive functioning (Keshavan et al., 2017). Another foundational proof-of-concept study by Wykes and colleagues found similar effects in fronto-cortical areas during cognitive remediation that was associated with improved memory function (Wykes et al., 2002). There have now emerged enough studies of the effects of cognitive training on brain function in schizophrenia to support a meta-analysis, in which the authors found consistent increases in activation in the prefrontal, medial temporal, and parietal cortices following cognitive remediation (Ramsay & MacDonald, 2015). Thus, there is growing evidence that cognitive enhancement interventions can shape the brain in schizophrenia in positive directions and that pre-treatment neural characteristics may significantly moderate response to such interventions.

8.8 Summary

- Schizophrenia is a heterogeneous condition for which response to cognitive enhancement interventions is variable.
- Cognitive enhancement is most suitable for patients who are symptomatically stable and have sufficient general intellectual ability to understand and benefit from treatment.
- Cognitive enhancement interventions are effective in both early course and long-term patients with schizophrenia and schizoaffective disorder, with additional functional benefits associated with early intervention; evidence is emerging on their efficacy in psychotic bipolar disorder.
- Biological markers to that index and moderate treatment outcomes are emerging and expected to be a significant focus of future research.

Choosing the Right Treatment for the Right Patient

9.1 Introduction

The science behind cognitive enhancement approaches in schizophrenia and related disorders indicates that cognitive training is generally effective for improving problems in processing speed, attention, memory, and the executive functions (McGurk et al., 2007b; Wykes et al., 2011). A smaller number of approaches are also effective for enhancing social cognition (Kurtz & Richardson, 2011), or the ability to process and interpret socioemotional information in oneself and others (Newman, 2001). Reading the literature on cognitive enhancement, the practitioner might mistakenly believe that all approaches are equally effective for all patients or that certain approaches can be applied broadly to the patient population without personalization to the unique needs and circumstances of the individual receiving the treatment. Although much of what is conducted in cognitive enhancement interventions can now be automated, particularly in those interventions that utilize computer-based approaches, the individuality and personal needs of patients living with schizophrenia necessitates that practitioners personalize their application of cognitive enhancement interventions for people living with schizophrenia and related disorders.

As reviewed in Chapter 8, there are numerous moderators of response to cognitive training. Further, there is at least as much heterogeneity in treatment approaches as there are in the populations of patients with schizophrenia, making the personalization of treatment to the range of circumstances faced by the patient exceedingly important for treatment engagement and success. Issues such as cognitive style, symptom stability, co-occurring substance use problems, and phase of illness are all personal characteristics with which each patient will present, that need to be considered when selecting the "right" cognitive enhancement approach. The use of bottom-up versus top-down training, whether to focus on social-cognitive abilities, and whether to use a targeted versus generalized training approach are all treatment factors that also vary across cognitive training programs. How then, is the practitioner to select the right treatment for the right patient in face of so many options and such patient heterogeneity? This chapter will illustrate, through a series of case examples, the application of evidence surrounding the moderators of response to cognitive training reviewed in Chapter 8 to personalize cognitive enhancement interventions to meet the unique needs and circumstances of a range of patients with schizophrenia.

9.2 Basics First

> **Case Study 9.1**
>
> John is a 22-year-old African American male who has been living with his grandmother since graduating high school. He developed schizoaffective disorder last year when he was 21, and he and his family have been struggling to cope with the condition ever since. He presents with a disorganized cognitive style, having difficulty focusing and paying attention for any significant length of time, and while his speech is somewhat organized, he often moves from topic to topic and it is difficult to follow his main point. His positive symptoms are mostly stable, but still quite severe, as John hears distressing voices every day and continues to withdraw from public situations due to high levels of paranoia.
>
> Recently, his family has become increasingly frustrated with John's behavior, as he has been staying out late, using drugs and alcohol, and forgetting to take his medicine. When John returns home in the evening after a long night out with his new girlfriend, he is often intoxicated, belligerent, paranoid about his family members, and destructive to his grandmother's property. John has difficulty managing his emotions, is fearful of the voices he is hearing, and believes going out on the town with his girlfriend is the only "normal" part of the life he has left.
>
> After several months of troubling behavior, John's grandmother indicates she can no longer care for him and he must find his own housing immediately. Now living on the streets with his girlfriend and sleeping at friends' houses when they can, John is running out of medication, does not have health insurance or money to pay for his antipsychotic treatment and other basic needs, and is having trouble finding a doctor who will see him without insurance. John has no income, no job, and no place to live. His cognitive challenges clearly play a role in his functional disability, as do his lack of financial resources, employment, and treatment providers.

John presents a situation that unfortunately is not uncommon for people living with schizophrenia, particularly young people who are struggling in their first several years of illness. His cognitive challenges in attention and organization are prominent and noticeable even to his family members, and clearly warrant treatment, as they make it difficult for him to organize his day, follow through on treatment recommendations, and maintain employment. Despite the prominence of John's cognitive challenges, his situation is an illustration of when a cognitive training specialist should be thinking of treatments other than cognitive enhancement to help John get back on his feet. John has numerous basic needs that must first be met before he can be reasonably referred to a cognitive training program. He is homeless, does not know where his next meal will come from, and is in significant need of basic treatment resources, such as a psychiatrist and medication. As long as these issues are outstanding, it will be extremely difficult for John to sit in front of a computer and complete cognitive training exercises to improve his attention and organization.

Cognitive enhancement approaches have grown significantly in popularity and application for patients with schizophrenia, but they are not a panacea. None of these cognitive enhancement interventions provide housing, food, medication, or any of the other primary needs with which John is struggling. John's case illustrates the importance of providing "basics first" to people living with schizophrenia and related conditions. Classically, Maslow identified a hierarchy of needs for human beings that indicated that primary needs must be met first before secondary and tertiary needs (Maslow, 1943). The same principle applies to the use of cognitive enhancement. Clear, organized thought and the absence of cognitive challenges is a human need for everyone, including those living with schizophrenia, but it is a distal need from the proximal needs of food, shelter, medicine and the like. John's immediate challenges are best addressed not through referral to a cognitive enhancement specialist, but to a service coordinator who can help find him affordable housing, help him to obtain disability benefits to pay for his housing, treatment and medication, and to help connect him again to effective psychiatric services. We have experience in attempting to include individuals experiencing the same challenges as John in cognitive enhancement programs. In the vast majority of situations, such individuals drop out of treatment in search of more practical help that will meet their basic needs. To maximize treatment retention and efficacy, it is therefore of paramount importance that the practitioner ensure basic needs are first met before offering cognitive training.

9.3 Psychiatric Stability

Case Study 9.2

Jane is a 40-year-old Caucasian woman who developed schizophrenia after college when she was 28. She has a husband, whom she has been married to since before she became ill, and together they have two children. Jane has had a difficult illness course, but with the help of clozapine, she has been able to gain good control over her positive symptoms. She continues to hear voices weekly, but not daily, and recognizes that they are part of her condition. She does not act on the voices she hears anymore, and while she continues to have some delusional thinking surrounding auditory hallucinations, she can reliably question whether her beliefs are true and often knows that her thinking is "paranoid" and not based on reality.

Jane has prominent negative symptoms that have been present since she developed the condition and are untreated. She presents with an unmotivated cognitive style, has difficulty using elaborated speech, often gives one-word answers, and experiences reduced processing speed and mental stamina. These cognitive challenges are making it difficult for Jane to find and maintain employment, which is personally important to her and her family. She has extreme difficulty during the interview process, often appearing flat and uninterested in the job, and on the job she experiences challenges keeping up with the fast pace and making friends with her co-workers.

Case Study 9.3

Mary is a 35-year-old Caucasian female who developed schizophrenia when she was 20. She is single and living with her parents, and she would very much like to move to her own apartment and gain greater independence in her life. Since the beginning of her condition, Mary has had very prominent positive symptoms, experiencing significant delusions of grandeur and persecution, which resulted in her hospitalization due to repeated public outbursts about being on a reality television show, ultimately leading her to break into the local television station to obtain her "footage."

Antipsychotic treatment has helped reduce these symptoms to some extent, but she continues to hear voices daily for most of the day and she believes that her psychiatrist may be involved in the reality television show in which she is starring. She is ambivalent about taking her antipsychotic medication, leading to variable adherence, and when she is under stress, her positive symptoms often become elevated to the point where an acute hospitalization seems imminent. Mary has an inflexible cognitive style, sticks to a rigid and limited routine, often has difficulty identifying alternative problem-solving strategies, is very nervous about ambiguity, and perseverates on topics of frustration.

The above examples present two very different cases of psychiatric and symptom stability, particularly with regard to positive symptoms. As reviewed in Chapter 8, positive symptom stability is a critical moderator of the efficacy of cognitive enhancement interventions, and those individuals with unstable positive symptoms experience less benefit from these interventions than individuals with stabilized positive symptoms (Wykes et al., 2011). What are the differences in this area that can be observed between Jane and Mary, and how do these differences reflect heterogeneity in their readiness for cognitive remediation? Jane clearly continues to experience positive symptoms, and the complete absence of such symptoms is not the criterion that the practitioner should be attempting to identify for cognitive training readiness. Despite continuing to experience positive symptoms on a weekly basis, the frequency is not daily, and most importantly, Jane has learned that her auditory hallucinations are a symptom of schizophrenia, not stimuli that are based in reality. This pattern of positive symptoms has been present and stable for the last 6 months, and Jane is adherent to her antipsychotic treatment to increase the likelihood that these symptoms remain under control. Jane's case illustrates a picture of positive symptom stability that is well-suited for beginning cognitive enhancement to address her cognitive challenges in processing speed, mental stamina, and elaboration. That she experiences significant and persistent negative symptoms is a concern for her care, but not an impediment to beginning cognitive training. In fact, some studies suggest that the treatment of cognitive impairments in schizophrenia may simultaneously address some aspects of negative symptom challenges (Eack et al., 2013). Further, the negative symptoms, while significant, are not so severe as to preclude her participation in the treatment. Consequently, the control Jane has been able to gain over her positive symptoms, while they are not completely remitted, will enable her to get more out of cognitive training than individuals who are still having difficulty with unstable positive symptoms.

Mary, on the other hand, presents with a concerning pattern of positive symptoms and medication ambivalence. The frequency of her positive symptoms is high: she usually experienced daily. Further, her insight into her condition is relatively low, as she continues to believe that some of her auditory hallucinations are evidence for her delusional beliefs of being a reality television star. The situation is further complicated by Mary being less adherent to her antipsychotic treatment, which only reduces its efficacy and heightens the challenge of stabilizing her positive symptoms. In addition, like so many other individuals with schizophrenia, stress plays a marked role in Mary's condition. She is highly vulnerable to stress, experiences stress from her positive symptoms, as well as her inability to live independently, which is personally important to her. Because of her cognitive inflexibility, however, Mary has great difficulty in changing her patterns of behavior, trying new strategies to manage stressful situations, and believing anything new could help her deal better with her positive symptoms.

The situation Mary is experiencing is unfortunately very common in schizophrenia. People with schizophrenia often get entrenched in their positive symptoms, which interfere with treatment, cause stress, and ultimately produce and maintain positive symptoms and delusional explanations for their existence. Cognitive training could begin, but Mary would likely benefit little from training exercises, and would probably become fixated on some aspect of the treatment that reinforces her delusional system of being a reality star. Her frequent auditory hallucinations would make it exceedingly difficult for her to engage in group or computer-based exercises. Paying attention, concentrating, completing difficult tasks, and other advanced cognitive functions are challenging enough for people living with the cognitive deficits associated with schizophrenia. Hearing voices regularly only makes these challenges more difficult, and suggests that cognitive enhancement is not the ideal next step in Mary's treatment. Interventions to enhance Mary's ability to consistently adhere to antipsychotic treatment and manage her stress would likely be much more effective at improving her course of illness than cognitive enhancement at this time, and may, in fact, help Mary progress to where she can be more likely to benefit from cognitive training interventions (see Chapter 4 for a discussion of approaches to stabilization of psychotic illness and Chapter 7 for optimum psychopharmacological management in an effort to enable readiness for cognitive enhancement).

9.4 Motivation and Engagement

Case Study 9.4

Paul is a 40-year-old African American male who has been living with schizophrenia since he was 19. He has had a difficult course with the illness, experiencing homelessness and disruptions related to substance use, when he was younger. After some years of attempting to stabilize his condition, he has found an antipsychotic medication that he likes and works well for him. He enjoys meeting with his psychiatrist, with whom he has an excellent therapeutic relationship, is open about his ongoing thoughts of the CIA tracking his behavior, and questions whether such symptoms are really true. Although Paul remains somewhat paranoid from time to time, his positive symptoms have largely stabilized, and he really would like to begin searching for a job.

Paul has a disorganized cognitive style that makes it difficult for him to pay attention at work or school, and he often gets lost in the details of tasks he needs to complete, rather than focusing on the main point or "gist" of his work goals. These cognitive challenges have resulted in Paul being relieved from his prior employment on several occasions, as he tends to fall behind others he is working with and is not able to complete the tasks relevant to his job on time.

Paul's therapist suggested cognitive remediation to address some of his challenges in organization and has referred him to the "Thinking Skills for Work" program (see Chapter 6 for review), an integrated cognitive training and supported employment program for people with schizophrenia and related conditions (McGurk et al., 2015). Paul appreciates the referral, but wants to get to work right away; after all, he has been out of the workforce for many years and does not want to lose any more time. He says to his therapist, "What are these computer games going to do for me? I don't need to play on the computer, I need to get back to work."

Paul's case presents a situation where cognitive enhancement could be quite helpful to his long-term goals of re-engaging in employment. However, Paul does not yet see the connection between his cognitive challenges and *his own* recovery goals. As a consequence, he is hesitant to begin a new treatment and wonders whether it will really help him achieve his vocational goals. Cognitive impairments associated with schizophrenia are commonly overlooked treatment targets by practitioners and patients alike. Because the positive symptoms of psychosis are the cardinal features of schizophrenia, and that effective treatments for remediating impairments in cognition have only recently emerged, many patients, and even their clinicians, do not often attend to the role of cognition in supporting personal recovery goals. At the onset of schizophrenia, the emphasis is appropriately on reducing psychotic symptoms, and in Paul's case, the challenges he has had in obtaining positive symptom stability have meant that his treatment has focused almost exclusively on reducing hallucinations and delusions. Now that such symptoms have come under good control, Paul naturally wonders why he has to undergo another treatment program to achieve his goals of returning to work, and how focusing on cognition is relevant to his recovery.

It is generally important for practitioners to assess and emphasize the role of cognitive challenges in achieving a meaningful functional recovery from schizophrenia. The emergence of a substantial evidence base supporting the efficacy of cognitive enhancement approaches in treating these deficits has generated substantial enthusiasm throughout the provider community, and conversations surrounding the role of social and non-social cognitive impairments in the course of schizophrenia and related conditions are now occurring with significantly greater frequency than ever before. However, this conversation has not been had with Paul, and prior to referring him to the Thinking Skills for Work Program, his clinician needs to engage Paul in a discussion about his cognitive style, and the role of disorganization in preventing him from reaching his work goals.

In referring patients to any new treatment approach, it is essential that the practitioner starts where the patient is in order to facilitate treatment engagement and motivation. Cognitive enhancement is no exception. Paul is currently excited about work, enthused about his recent symptom recovery from schizophrenia, and at the same time is unaware that his cognitive challenges are likely to present barriers to his recovery goals. Rather than beginning with a referral to the Thinking Skills for Work Program, the practitioner must engage Paul in a dialog surrounding his recovery goals and factors that may impact them. A central part of this conversation would be a discussion of Paul's disorganized cognitive style, and guided reflection on how his thinking has produced challenges with employment in the past. In this way, the connection between organized thinking and work success can begin to emerge in Paul's own assessment of his strengths and challenges.

Many patients do not recognize that they experience significant cognitive challenges associated with their condition, and the connection between these impairments and recovery goals is not often a focus of treatment discussions. Like any other psychological treatment, motivation and engagement are essential factors in successful completion of treatment and achievement of the desired response. Paul's case illustrates the importance of having clear discussions with patients surrounding their cognitive strengths and weaknesses, in order to raise awareness of these issues as important factors in their treatment and recovery. Paul's case also underscores the importance of connecting cognitive challenges to larger functional goals. If the practitioner can help Paul make the connection between more organized thinking and work readiness and success, Paul will be much more likely to engage in the Thinking Skills for Work Program and be motivated to put effort into his participation. One of the most consistent themes we have observed in clinical practice is that the more patients put into their participation in cognitive enhancement approaches, the more likely they are to obtain meaningful benefits from their efforts. As such, it is essential for the practitioner to connect cognition with personal recovery goals, and for treatment conversations to extend beyond the management of positive symptoms.

By starting where the person is and drawing these connections between cognition and functioning, patients will become more motivated to engage in cognitive training and ultimately be more likely to experience its benefits.

9.5 Bottom-Up versus Top-Down Training

Case Study 9.5

Tom is a 22-year-old Caucasian male who recently developed schizoaffective disorder. His positive and mood symptoms have been well-controlled with antipsychotic and mood stabilizer medications, but he continues to have tremendous difficulty in problem-solving, planning, and developing strategies to address even the most basic tasks required for his daily functioning. He has difficulty organizing his day, keeping track of his group home chores, and attending treatment appointments. He often shows up to the clinic on the wrong day, and when he is scheduled to see a member of service team, Tom is usually absent or arrives quite late. Tom and his therapist have been discussing the difficulties he has been having in his day-to-day life, and the role that cognitive challenges in executive function, and strategic thinking, have in his problems with attending treatment appointments and completing activities required for his daily living.

Case Study 9.6

Chi is a 25-year-old Asian female who also recently developed schizoaffective disorder. Like Tom, Chi has had good success in stabilizing her psychotic and mood symptoms with medication treatment. However, she continues to have great difficulty in processing information quickly. Chi usually takes several seconds to respond to a question, despite near-complete reduction of auditory hallucinations since she began antipsychotic treatment. Chi's movement is significantly slowed, her body language is impoverished, and while she can problem-solve through most challenging situations, it takes her a great deal of time to arrive at a solution. Her mental stamina is reduced, and Chi has significant difficulty in keeping up with conversations. Chi and her therapist have been discussing her reduced mental stamina and slowed processing, and believe these factors are a significant impediment to her success in college, where she hopes to return soon.

Tom and Chi present with two prototypically different cognitive styles. Tom has extensive challenges with higher-order thinking and executive functioning, which manifest as difficulty in problem-solving, planning, and strategic thinking. Chi, on the other hand, is significantly "slowed down" by her cognitive challenges, and experiences delays in processing and interpreting information. Neuropsychological testing using the MATRICS Consensus Cognitive Battery (Green et al., 2004) reveals a different profile of cognitive impairments for Chi and Tom (see Table 9.1).

Tom has normal attention and speed of processing, but significant impairments in working memory, problem-solving, and verbal learning, which extend to social cognition. Chi has excellent working memory and above-average problem-solving abilities, but significantly impaired speed of processing and attention, which extends to visual

Table 9.1 Neuropsychological testing results for Tom and Chi using the MATRICS consensus Cognitive Battery

	Tom	Chi
Domain	Percentile (%)	Percentile (%)
Speed of processing	50	10
Attention/vigilance	52	5
Working memory	20	75
Visual learning and memory	30	20
Verbal learning and memory	15	50
Reasoning and problem-solving	10	60
Social cognition	25	40

learning. Chi's social-cognitive impairments are present, but not as great in magnitude as those experienced by Tom. These two cognitive profiles suggest different approaches to cognitive enhancement.

Given the processing speed and attention impairments experienced by Chi, a bottom-up approach to cognitive training is likely to be more helpful than a top-down approach. As reviewed previously in Chapter 4, bottom-up approaches to cognitive enhancement are those that focus on improving early signal processing and basic, lower-order cognitive abilities, such as attention and processing speed. The underlying premise behind such approaches is that information is entering the brain in a "noisy" fashion, which delays processing and makes it difficult to attend to specific stimuli. Numerous studies have documented these challenges in the visual and auditory systems of patients with schizophrenia (Erickson, Ruffle, & Gold, 2016). brainHQ by Posit Science is one example of a bottom-up cognitive training approach that seeks to increase auditory signal processing through repeated practice of auditory discrimination tasks, which have been shown to enhance auditory processing and other aspects of cognition (Fisher et al., 2009). This approach is likely to be most appropriate for Chi, and through addressing her basic impairments in attention and processing speed, further benefits are likely to be observed in memory, problem-solving, and social cognition.

Given the pattern of higher-order impairments in reasoning and problem-solving that Tom experiences, a top-down approach to cognitive enhancement is likely to be more effective for him. Top-down approaches focus on addressing higher-order executive function skills first, suggesting that lower-order difficulties in basic memory and learning, are the result of disorganized planning, problem-solving, and strategic thinking (see Chapter 4 for review). Using PSSCogRehab by Bracy is one potential cognitive enhancement approach for Tom, where he can work on higher-order problem-solving tasks that require him to plan ahead and develop strategies to complete the training exercises. Through developing better problem-solving abilities, Tom is also likely to improve his other executive challenges in working memory, as well as his impairments in social cognition.

Tom and Chi illustrate the diversity of cognitive challenges patients with schizophrenia and related disorders can experience. In the face of such heterogeneity, the practitioner must be mindful that different approaches to cognitive enhancement are designed to address different impairments in cognition. While evidence is not yet available on the comparative efficacy of bottom-up versus top-down training approaches, the nature of cognitive challenges patients experience often point to specific approaches that are likely to be most helpful. For those individuals who experience deficits in lower-order cognitive abilities, such as attention and processing speed, a bottom-up approach is thought to be more effective. For people experiencing higher-order challenges in executive functioning, planning, and problem-solving, a top-down approach that directly addresses these deficits has been viewed as more appropriate.

It is important to recognize that the cognitive profile in schizophrenia is not often as distinct as what is presented in Tom and Chi's cases. Often a combination of higher-order and lower-order impairments are present. There appears to be far more evidence for a generalized cognitive deficit in schizophrenia that affects many domains, rather than an isolated profile of cognitive challenges (Dickinson et al., 2008), which suggests that practitioners need to be prepared to handle multiple types of lower- and higher-order cognitive challenges in patients with schizophrenia and related disorders. A comprehensive neuropsychological assessment, such as provided by the MATRICS Battery, can help identify the specific cognitive needs of each patient, so that the practitioner can recommend the appropriate approach to cognitive enhancement, whether it be bottom-up training, top-down training, or a combination of the two.

9.6 Personalizing Treatment Protocols

In order to optimize the efficacy of cognitive enhancement and to facilitate treatment engagement, it is essential that cognitive training models tailor their approaches to the goals, strengths, and challenges of the patient. Paul's case example above illustrates the importance of linking cognitive enhancement strategies to meaningful functional goals to enhance motivation (e.g. emphasizing how improving his organization will help Paul maintain employment). Such linkage to functional and recovery goals is important, however, not just for improving motivation, but also for improving broader functional outcomes. A critical element of effective cognitive enhancement is a growing awareness on the part of the patient (and oftentimes the clinician) of how cognitive challenges present barriers to recovery and the achievement of life goals. When individuals become aware of their cognitive challenges and the role they play in contributing to disability, many become motivated to address those issues and the practitioner and patient often become aware of the cognitive elements that are particularly affecting the patient's personal goals. This increased awareness of the link between cognition and functioning helps the practitioner to tailor cognitive exercises and coaching strategies to those that are most related to the patient's functional goals. These goals will of course be different for every patient, making the personalization and tailoring of treatment an important part of the effective practice of cognitive enhancement.

There are numerous methods of tailoring cognitive enhancement approaches to the patient. Some programs use remarkably little tailoring, and provide standardized training across a diverse array of patients. Other programs focus on tailoring cognitive exercises to the neuropsychology of the patient, often in an automated fashion based on either a set of assessments or cognitive task performance. This latter approach can be helpful in making cognitive enhancement protocols more efficient, by targeting them to the specific deficits experienced by each patient. However, these approaches, while efficient, under-emphasize the connection between cognitive training and patient functioning. Such approaches also often rely on specialized cognitive training software, such as brainHQ (see Chapter 5), that is not available in other training packages. Development of a *Recovery Plan* is a third approach to the personalization of cognitive training that is employed in Cognitive Enhancement Therapy (CET; Hogarty & Greenwald, 2006), and is widely applicable to many different cognitive enhancement approaches.

A Recovery Plan in CET is a brief plan that outlines the primary goal of the patient for cognitive training, the cognitive challenge he or she is experiencing that is presenting a barrier to that goal, and a set of strategies the patient can use to help address the cognitive challenge and facilitate the achievement of his or her goal. The basic structure of a recovery plan is outlined in Box 9.1.

In the Recovery Plan, the practitioner must be careful to select goals that are meaningful to the patient and also goals that can be realistically tied to cognitive impairment and accomplished during the course of the cognitive training program. As such, the nature of the goal will be adapted, in part, to the length of the program. Relatively short-term programs that last for 10–12 weeks would more profitably focus on short-term goals, such as improving organization, improving attention, and increasing social contacts. Longer-term programs, such as CET, which is provided over the course of 18 months, can more realistically focus on longer-term goals, such as school and work. However, even 18 months is a fairly short period to get back into school and work for some individuals, and the practitioner should be careful to select a goal with the patient that can be reasonably accomplished within the time frame of the intervention. Goal selection should be a collaborative discussion between the patient, clinician, and family, if available. Shared decision-making is an important part of patient engagement, and if the clinician only selects goals that he feels the patient needs, but the patient does not agree or see the importance of these goals, outcomes from treatment are likely to be limited (see Chapter 4).

The problem selected should be one or two presenting cognitive issues that are clearly tied to the achievement of the goal. For example, if the goal is focused on going back to school and the patient is having trouble paying attention, difficulty in maintaining attention would likely be the problem of focus. Often, patients have multiple problems that are barriers to achieving their goals. Multiple problems can be listed, but the practitioner

---

Box 9.1 Structure of a personalized recovery plan in Cognitive Enhancement Therapy

Goal: A goal that is related to cognitive impairment that the patient can realistically work toward during the time frame of the cognitive training program

   Problem: The primary cognitive problem (or two) that is a barrier to the achievement of the goal

Strategies:

1. A list of strategies the patient can use to address the problem and achieve their goal.
2. Strategies often include participation in cognitive training.
3. Strategies also often include activities and exercises the patient can perform outside of cognitive training to promote application and generalization.
4. Many strategies also focus on stress management, exercise, and other basic psychological techniques that can be used to improve cognition, beyond cognitive training.

must be careful not to work on more problems than is feasible during the course of treatment. In our experience, working on more than two or three presenting problems simultaneously tends to be less feasible, even with longer cognitive enhancement programs.

Finally, after the goal and presenting problem(s) are identified, the patient and practitioner work to select some strategies that will be used to address the problem(s) and help the patient achieve their goal. These strategies not only often include participation in cognitive training exercises, but also usually enumerate strategies in everyday life that can be taken to improve thinking and cognition. Such strategies commonly include exercise, a healthy sleep routine, engaging in more frequent social contacts, and relaxation methods, all of which can impact cognition. The practitioner must be careful to identify strategies beyond cognitive training that patients can use in their daily lives to enhance their cognition, and application of strategies learned during training, in order to promote generalization and improve functioning beyond performance in the more controlled therapeutic context. Box 9.2 provides some examples of recovery plans for different goals and cognitive challenges that the practitioner can use to help guide the collaborative development of recovery plans with their own patients.

9.7 What Specific Treatment Do I Choose?

In schizophrenia, there now exist over 40 randomized-controlled trials of cognitive enhancement approaches. While the evidence suggests that, on average, these approaches are helpful for improving cognition, functioning, and to some degree psychopathology, there are nearly as many different types of cognitive training programs as there are studies that make up the evidence base. This situation has made it exceedingly difficult for practitioners and policymakers to identify which cognitive training approach is most appropriate, effective, and beneficial for particular patients or populations. The current state of the evidence base does not have a clear answer to the question: "What cognitive enhancement approach works for whom?" One could examine effect sizes from the latest meta-analytic reviews (McGurk et al., 2007b; Wykes et al., 2011) and identify the treatments with the largest effect size and smallest standard error. Such a survey would identify brainHQ, Cogpack, and CET as some of the most reliably effective cognitive training programs for schizophrenia, but this would also require comparisons across very different treatment protocols, treatment durations, and patient characteristics. Without a head-to-head comparisons using standardized treatment protocols and patient inclusion criteria, it is exceedingly difficult to compare the efficacy of interventions across heterogenous clinical trials.

At this time, perhaps the most profitable way to select a cognitive training intervention for implementation or patient referral is to consider the presenting needs of the particular patient. Does the patient have a limited set of cognitive challenges that primarily represent difficulties in neurocognition? If so, a program that provides only neurocognitive training may be most beneficial and efficient. Does the patient present with predominantly higher-order cognitive dysfunction in planning, problem-solving, and organization? A top-down training approach, such as PSSCogRehab may be most helpful in such cases. Does the patient present with a greater number of lower-order cognitive challenges in attention and processing speed? A bottom-up training approach, such as brainHQ may be most effective. Does the patient have significant social impairment

---

Box 9.2 Example recovery plans from Cognitive Enhancement Therapy that personalize cognitive training

Example A

Goal: To improve my attention during conversations

Problem: Difficulty maintaining attention/easily distracted

Strategies: 1. Cue myself to pay attention.
                        2. Take notes in the CET group to avoid distraction.
                        3. Actively listen and ask questions in conversations.
                        4. Focus on the gist when talking with others.
                        5. Paraphrase back to the other person in conversations.
                        6. Use computer training to boost attention.

Example B

Goal: To improve my performance at work

Problem: Difficulty with motivation, feeling slowed down

Strategies: 1. Develop a daily sleep schedule and stick to it.
                        2. Volunteer to be the chairperson in CET group.
                        3. Increase processing speed through computer training.
                        4. Breaking assignments down in small parts.
                        5. Reward myself when I succeed at work.
                        6. Talk to my doctor to see if my medication dose can be adjusted.

Example C

Goal: To increase my network of friends

Problem: Having a small social network

Strategies: 1. Assess situations to decide who I want to get to know further. Work on initiating and maintaining conversations.
                        2. Use CET strategies: active listening, perspective taking, foresightfulness, social context appraisal.
                        3. Make an effort to know new people while keeping up with current friends.
                        4. Use humor in conversations. Try to be less serious and more relaxed. Coach myself using positive self-talk.
                        5. Express myself more to others – use elaborated speech.

Source: Adapted from Eack (2012), reprinted with permission.

---

and challenges in understanding and processing socio-emotional information? An intervention that integrated neurocognitive and social-cognitive training, such as CET, may be the most optimal approach in such cases. The practitioner can use the treatments reviewed in Chapters 5 and 6 to inform herself of the different cognitive enhancement approaches and their foci, and should match these to the needs of the patient based on presenting problems, neuropsychological assessment, and other available data.

Finally, given the emerging nature of cognitive enhancement in community treatment settings, feasibility may be the most significant criterion upon which to base treatment referrals for cognitive enhancement. Most states are fortunate if they have implemented any cognitive training approach, let alone multiple different options to meet the needs of a diverse patient population. In a majority of situations, the practitioner will only have available a single treatment approach within their catchment area, and that will be the approach selected, even if not a perfect fit for the needs of the patient. When considering implementation, feasibility is also a significant factor, as many agencies do not have the capacity to implement more comprehensive programs without additional funding or reimbursement, leaving more targeted and less integrated treatment options as the most feasible. Practitioners, policy makers, patients, and family members will need to advocate for the routine integration of effective cognitive enhancement programs, as such interventions currently lack reimbursement codes or are not covered by many states. In the future, it is hoped that more evidence will be generated around what specific treatment should be provided to each patient, but in the meantime, the practitioner will need to select a cognitive training approach that is evidence-based, targeted to the needs of the patient, and feasible.

9.8 Summary

- Cognitive enhancement is not a first-line treatment for schizophrenia and related disorders, and practitioners should ensure that basic needs are met, and psychotic symptoms are stabilized, before beginning cognitive training.
- Currently, the selection of different cognitive enhancement approaches is based on feasibility, availability, and patient need; future research will need to generate head-to-head comparisons of different training approaches to identify for whom specific treatments are most effective.
- Regardless of the cognitive enhancement approach selected, it is essential that goals are developed collaboratively with the patient and that a clear connection is made between cognitive challenges and personal recovery goals.
- Approaches to cognitive enhancement should be personalized to the unique needs of the patient, and Recovery Plans can be an effective method for such personalization.

Chapter 10

Approaches to Assessment and Monitoring Treatment Response

10.1 Introduction

Personalizing and optimizing cognitive enhancement approaches for patients with schizophrenia and related disorders involves tailoring training methods and parameters to the unique needs and goals of the individual, and understanding how personal cognitive and clinical factors impact treatment selection and response. Furthermore, with the implementation of any new treatment approach, good clinical practice indicates that it is essential to monitor its impact on patient outcomes, even outside the context of a research study. Effective cognitive and clinical assessment is at the core of understanding patient factors for treatment selection and personalization, as well as evaluating the impact of cognitive enhancement interventions. Much of what has been described in Chapters 8 and 9 to personalize treatment to the unique circumstances of the individual patient relies heavily on prior assessment data. Whether a bottom-up or top-down training approach is appropriate depends upon understanding the degree of lower-order and higher-order cognitive impairments experienced not by the population of patients with schizophrenia in general, but by the individual patient sitting in your office awaiting treatment. Additionally, tailoring cognitive enhancement and developing individualized recovery plans relies upon collaborative discussion and data collection between the practitioner and patient to understand the most pressing cognitive issues and how they contribute to meaningful functional goals for the patient. The collection of such data may seem esoteric outside of research settings, but the best clinical practice models indicate that assessment should be an ongoing, continuous part of the implementation of novel interventions. Approaches to overall clinical and cognitive assessment are outlined in Chapter 4. This chapter will review assessment tools that community practitioners outside of research settings can use to assess the cognitive strengths and challenges of the patients they seek to help, as well as instruments practitioners can utilize to monitor cognitive, clinical, and functional responses to cognitive training.

10.2 Standardized Neuropsychological Assessments

The research evidence for cognitive enhancement has largely relied upon standardized neuropsychological tests that have been used in practice for decades. These tests are reviewed extensively in Chapter 1 in the discussion of assessing cognition, and include the Wechsler Adult Intelligence Scales (Wechsler, 1981), the Wisconsin Card Sorting Test (Heaton et al., 1993), Trails A and B (War Department, Adjutant General's Office [Army Individual Test Battery, 1944]), and other common standard neuropsychological assessments. These tests require extensive training and administration by a psychological testing professional, usually a doctoral-level psychologist, making them excellent measures for research settings, but less ideal for community practice where reliably trained psychologists may not be as readily available. For those agencies that have testing resources, the MATRICS Consensus Cognitive Battery (Green et al., 2004) is an excellent option for standardized neuropsychological assessment, in that it combines some of the most reliable and relevant cognitive tests for schizophrenia into a single assessment battery. This battery is now the field standard assessment for cognitive enhancement interventions in research, and settings with the resources to administer the MATRICS Battery will find it is a valuable tool for cognitive characterization and monitoring treatment response. We also recommend the use of the full Mayer-Salovey-Caruso Emotional Intelligence Test (MSCEIT; Mayer et al., 2003) to supplement the rather limited social-cognitive assessment provided by the MATRICS Battery. Standardized self-administered cognitive assessments, such as the Penn Computerized Neurocognitive Battery (Gur et al., 2010) are also good options when testing resources are limited, but continue to rely upon neuropsychology professionals for setup and interpretation. When an agency has sufficient access to psychologists and testing staff, the use of standardized neuropsychological assessments to monitor treatment progress during cognitive enhancement is highly recommended.

10.3 Practitioner-Friendly Measures of Cognitive Change

Many medium- and smaller-sized agencies do not have doctoral-level psychologists on staff or other professionals qualified to administer standardized neuropsychological tests. In such cases, assessment should *not* be abandoned. The practitioner will be "flying blind" without an adequate understanding of the patient's cognitive needs, and will not know when to try a different treatment approach or when to conclude training due to sufficient cognitive response. The absence of testing staff, however, means that agencies will need to turn to more practitioner-friendly assessments of cognitive ability. These assessments have received far less psychometric evaluation than those included in the MATRICS Consensus Cognitive Battery, and are likely to be less reliable and valid indicators of cognitive ability. They should not be used for diagnostics or serious clinical evaluation, but can be very helpful in obtaining a rapid and general understanding of a patient's cognitive abilities.

One measure that we have repeatedly found to be helpful in both research and clinical practice is the Cognitive Styles and Social Cognition Eligibility Interview (Hogarty et al., 2004), which is included in Appendix A of the Cognitive Enhancement Therapy training manual by Hogarty and Greenwald (2006), see www.CognitiveEnhancementTherapy .com. This measure consists of a 45 minute to 1 hour structured interview that provides an assessment of the patient's cognitive style (unmotivated, disorganized, or rigid) and social-cognitive challenges indicative of a need for treatment. In this interview, a clinically trained interviewer, usually a master's-level clinician who need not be a psychologist, takes the patient through a series of questions to generate responses the interviewer can use to rate the cognitive style and challenges of the patient. For example, the interview asks the patient, "How is your energy level? How many hours do you rest or sleep each day?" These questions are part of the interview assessing the unmotivated cognitive style, and a patient who responds that she is experiencing a low level of energy and sleeping 12–14 hours a day, including naps, would suggest a potentially low level of motivation and mental stamina. Through a series of such interview questions, the interviewer gathers information surrounding each of the three cognitive styles and then provides ratings on criteria for these styles. After completing the interview and associated rating form, the clinician will have available independent scores for each cognitive style and be able to determine which style is most prominent to guide treatment planning and implementation for that particular patient. Similar information is provided for social-cognitive challenges. The ease of access to and administration of the Cognitive Styles and Social Cognition Eligibility Interview makes it a good potential option for community settings that do not have the staffing resources for standardized neuropsychological testing.

As initially presented in Chapter 1, the Brief Assessment of Cognition in Schizophrenia is an excellent alternative performance-based measure of neurocognitive ability to the MATRICS Consensus Cognitive Battery for time-pressed practitioners with limited training. This battery is significantly shorter that the MATRICS battery, requiring approximately 30 minutes to administer and covering such cognitive domains as processing speed, verbal learning and memory, working memory, and executive functioning (Keefe, 2004). The measure was originally designed as a paper-and-pencil test, and has been widely validated in this modality. A computerized table-based version, the BAC App has also been developed, which significantly aids the administration of the battery and has convergence with the standard paper-and-pencil version of the test (Atkins et al., 2017).

For practitioners who are not able to administer performance-based assessments of cognitive ability, another brief interview-based assessment that has been developed and validated for patients with schizophrenia is the Schizophrenia Cognition Rating Scale (SCORS; Keefe et al., 2006). This 20-item interview-based measure, like the Cognitive Styles and Social Cognition Eligibility Interview, asks patients a series of questions related to their cognitive ability. For example, "Do you have difficulty with remembering names of people you know?" Questions a broad set of cognitive domains, including both social and non-social cognition, and largely correspond to those assessed in the MATRICS battery. The interview takes approximately 12 minutes to complete and 1–2 minutes to score, and ideally includes interviews with both the patient and a family member or other person who has regular contact with the patient (Keefe et al., 2006). Studies of the SCORS have demonstrated its convergence with performance-based measures, as well as its predictive association with functional outcome in patients with schizophrenia (Keefe et al., 2006).

Finally, a less brief, but easy-to-administer performance-based battery of cognitive assessments can be found in the Penn Computerized Neurocognitive Battery (Gur et al., 2010). This battery uses non-standardized neuropsychological tasks presented on the computer to assess attention, memory, spatial ability, motor speed, language, cognitive flexibility, and emotion processing. Certain tests can be selected out of the battery if the practitioner seeks to target specific domains. A particularly unique aspect of the Penn battery is its comprehensive assessment of emotion processing via three different emotion perception-related tests, providing greater coverage of this area of social cognition than most other validated neurocognitive batteries. The full Penn battery can take an hour or more to complete in patients with schizophrenia, however brief batteries have also been developed focused on memory, executive functioning, and emotion processing, most of which can be completed within 30 minutes. One of the most significant advantages of the

Penn battery is that it is computerized and largely self-administered, markedly reducing tester and administrator training and burden. Patients can easily complete the battery with little instruction and scores are automatically calculated for the practitioner.

With regard to social cognition, the full MSCEIT (Mayer et al., 2003) is an excellent option that we have previously observed to be psychometrically valid and sensitive to change in patients with schizophrenia (Eack et al., 2007, 2010). The MSCEIT is a lengthy (20–60 minutes) social-cognitive assessment of emotional intelligence, covering the emotion-processing domains of emotion perception, facilitation, understanding, and management (Salovey & Mayer, 1990). The MSCEIT is performance-based, in that it asks participants to solve emotion problems (e.g. match an emotion label to a face, identify the best strategy to manage an emotional state) rather than relying on self-report, and the managing emotions subscale of the measure has been included in the MATRICS Consensus Cognitive Battery (Green et al., 2004). Although the MSCEIT is not a brief measure, it is very practitioner-friendly, as it is primarily self-administered via the computer. Patients complete the test online, which generates normative scores on an intelligence metric (mean of 100, standard deviation of 15) for the practitioner to review and use in treatment planning or monitor social-cognitive change. The MSCEIT has been widely used and validated in schizophrenia research and offers a unique, performance-based assessment of social cognition not commonly addressed by other batteries.

In addition to the MSCEIT, there are a variety of other measures of social cognition that are easy for the practitioner to administer. Within the Penn Computerized Neurocognitive Battery (Gur et al., 2010), there exists a set of computer-based assessments of emotion processing, including the Penn Emotion Recognition Test (Kohler et al., 2003), which has been widely used in social-cognitive research with people with schizophrenia. This assessment takes 10–15 minutes to complete, is fully automated in administration via the computer, and will provide additional information on the ability of individuals to understand and identify emotional labels in human faces, a common problem for people with schizophrenia. To obtain assessments outside the emotion-processing domain, practitioners can utilize the Social Cognition Profile (Hogarty et al., 2004), which is a clinician-rated measure of behaviors indicative of adult social cognition originally developed for use with Cognitive Enhancement Therapy. The Social Cognition Profile has received less psychometric evaluation than other field standard measures of social cognition in schizophrenia, but is readily available in the CET manual (see Appendix D from Hogarty & Greenwald, 2006), is easy to administer, and covers a broad array of social-cognitive constructs, from perspective-taking to providing support to foresightfulness. Another novel measure of social cognition is the Relationships Across Domains (RAD) measure (Sergi et al., 2009), which consists of a series of vignettes that describe relationships between two individuals. After each vignette, respondents are asked a series of questions about whether certain behavior from one of the two individuals is characteristic of their relationship with the other, based on the information presented in the scenario. Using this approach, the RAD obtains information about whether participants understand social relationships and different relationship models presented in the task, making the RAD a unique assessment of social-cognitive ability distinct from other commonly used measures. The instrument is longer, taking approximately 35 minutes to complete, and requires sufficient reading ability, but is largely self-administered, making it easy to adopt for practitioners.

10.4 Assessing Functional Outcome and "Real World" Change

Measurement of change during the course of cognitive enhancement should not stop at the assessment of cognition, as patients, family members, and practitioners all are interested in functioning in the "real world" beyond what can be obtained via neuropsychological tests. Recall from Chapter 3 that cognitive enhancement is but a means to an end, and that cognition is targeted as an approach to improve functional recovery in patients with schizophrenia and related conditions. Consequently, in addition to measuring cognitive change, it is essential that practitioners also obtain an assessment of functional change during the course of treatment. There are many validated measures of patient functioning available in the literature, and some agencies already have specific measures implemented within their routine practice. For such situations, it is recommended that the practitioner rely upon the existing assessment infrastructure to monitor functional change, as this will provide a historical baseline from prior ratings and ease the assessment burden on patients and practitioners.

For settings that do not have a functional outcome measurement strategy in place, a brief assessment that includes both the patient and collateral (e.g. clinician, family member) perspective is recommended. Prior studies have shown that self-report ratings of functioning are less valid than those that are buttressed by clinical or family informants (Sabbag et al., 2011). One simple and very brief measure of functional outcome is the Global Assessment of Functioning (GAF; American Psychiatric Association, 2013) scale, which rates patient functioning (and symptomatology) in a 100-point scale, with higher scores representing better functioning. This measure is quick, commonly available, and often already in widespread use in routine clinical practice due to its inclusion in DSM-IV. The GAF is simple and easy to administer, but is less reliable and valid than other functional outcome assessments, so the accuracy and stability of data obtained from the measure can be limited. The practitioner will have to balance the limitations of this measure with its advantages, primarily in simplicity and speed, in determining whether it is appropriate for monitoring the functioning of their patients.

Another brief measure of patient functioning is the WHOQOL-BREF (World Health Organization, 1996), a brief version of the World Health Organization's quality of life scale that covers functioning in the areas physical health, psychological health, social relationships, and the environment. The WHOQOL-BREF is a self-report measure, and therefore a subjective assessment of quality of life, that has received extensive validation in the literature (Skevington, Lotfy, & O'Connell, 2004). The measure consists of 26 items rated on a 5-point scale, with higher scores indicating better perceived quality of life, and takes 15–20 minutes to complete, depending on the patient. Scores are manually calculated from online scoring documentation for the practitioner to use to monitor change in each of the domains of quality of life assessed by the instrument. Because the WHOQOL-BREF is a self-report measure, it is recommended that it be used in conjunction with another measure of patient functioning that obtains collateral information, so that multiple perspectives on the patient's functional ability can be obtained for a more comprehensive assessment of functional recovery and quality of life.

The Specific Levels of Functioning Scale (SLOF; Schneider & Struening, 1983) provides a comprehensive assessment of collateral (e.g. family, caregiver, clinician) perspectives on patient functioning in the areas of physical functioning, personal care, social functioning, activities of daily living, and work. The SLOF is an ideal instrument to pair with self-report measures because of its focus on collateral informants, such as the clinician, and consists of 43 items rated on a 5-point scale, with higher scores indicative of better functioning. The measure has been routinely used in schizophrenia research studies over the past decade, and has been identified as one of the top-rated measures of functional outcome by a RAND panel of experts in the area (Leifker et al., 2009). The SLOF is a longer measure, due to the greater number of domains it assesses, and takes approximately 20 minutes to complete. For other available measures of functional outcome, it is recommended that practitioners review the findings of the Validation of Everyday Real-World Outcomes (VALERO) study to identify those measures that are reliable, valid, and usable in everyday practice (e.g. Harvey et al., 2011; Leifker et al., 2009).

10.5 Monitoring Clinical Outcomes

Assessments of clinical status, including positive, negative, and general psychopathology symptoms, may not be obvious measures for inclusion in cognitive training programs, but there are a number of reasons why it may be important to track clinical outcomes during the course of cognitive enhancement. First, prior meta-analytic evidence does indicate a modest, but significant impact on positive symptoms associated with cognitive enhancement (McGurk et al., 2007b; Wykes et al., 2011). Second, the same meta-analytic evidence suggests that patients who start treatment with greater positive symptoms have less cognitive benefit associated with cognitive training (Wykes et al., 2011). Third, as reviewed in Chapter 8, symptom stability is an important eligibility criterion for inclusion in cognitive enhancement programs. Finally, it is often important for the practitioner to monitor symptom stability to determine if any true cognitive change has taken place during the course of treatment. Cognition can vary according to clinical state, depending on the domain (e.g. Herbener et al., 2005), and changes in positive symptoms due to medication or other changes can be reflected in repeated cognitive assessments. In order to avoid this "pseudospecificity," practitioners must monitor clinical status and evaluate cognitive change in conjunction with any corresponding clinical changes that might be occurring. As a consequence, it is often important to initially assess clinical symptoms, and because of the potential impact of cognitive training on symptom domains, it may also be beneficial for the practitioner to monitor symptom status throughout the course of treatment.

Brief symptom batteries are plentiful in schizophrenia research. One commonly used measure is the Brief Psychiatric Rating Scale (BPRS; Overall & Gorham, 1962), which consists of 18–24 items (depending on the version) that the clinician or interviewer uses to rate a broad set of psychiatric symptoms, ranging from positive symptoms to negative symptoms to those associated with depression and/or anxiety. The BPRS is one of the most widely used clinical assessments of psychiatric symptomatology in mental health and schizophrenia research (Faustman & Overall, 1999). The interview-based measure takes approximately 15–30 minutes to complete, and it is recommended that practitioners use the anchored version to increase the reliability of their ratings (Ventura et al., 1993). Items are rated on a 7-point scale from not present (1) to extremely severe (7), and ratings are based upon both interview questions and observational data collected during the interview. Because of the brief nature of the BPRS, its coverage of any single domain of psychopathology (e.g. positive symptoms) is limited to a few items, which can hamper more in-depth assessment of individual clinical domains. As a measure to monitor general clinical outcomes and eligibility for cognitive enhancement, however, the BPRS is a very good fit for hurried practitioners interested in obtaining reliable assessments of clinical psychopathology.

For greater depth in assessment of positive and negative symptoms, the Scale for Assessment of Positive Symptoms (SAPS; Andreasen, 1984) and the Scale for Assessment of Negative Symptoms (SANS; Andreasen, 1983) are two measures that provide reliable and valid assessments of these domains. Both the SAPS and the SANS are interview-based measures like the BPRS and should not be completed as a self-report measure. The SAPS consists of 34 items of specific positive symptoms rated on a 6-point scale ranging from none (0) to severe (5). The SANS consists of 25 items of specific negative symptoms (including some cognitive symptoms), also rated on the same 6-point metric as the SAPS. Combined, the two measures could take up to 120 minutes to complete, and while they represent gold standard measures of positive and negative symptomatology in the field, they may be more comprehensive than is needed for simply monitoring clinical status during cognitive enhancement. Recently, the Brief Negative Symptom Scale (Kirkpatrick et al., 2010) has been created to provide an updated and briefer assessment of negative symptoms in schizophrenia, which can be used instead of the SANS. This measure consists of 13 items rated on a 7-point scale from normal (0) to extremely severe (6), takes approximately 15 minutes to complete, and has shown significant convergence with the SANS. Unfortunately, there is not currently a corresponding brief measure of positive symptoms, and for such an assessment, it is recommended that practitioners use the BPRS.

For particularly hurried practitioners who do not need a granular level assessment of symptomatology, but merely want to monitor overall clinical status, the Clinical Global Impression Scale (CGI; Guy, 1976) is a quick and easy-to-use measure of overall clinical status. The CGI consists of two items, one focused on severity of illness and the other focused on clinical improvement. The CGI severity scale is likely to be the most useful for pre-treatment or eligibility screening and consists of a single item asking the practitioner to rate the severity of the patient's mental health condition on a 7-point scale from normal (1) to extremely ill (7). The CGI improvement scale is likely to be more useful for monitoring clinical change, and similar to the severity scale, asks the practitioner to rate the degree of clinical change since a given baseline (e.g. since starting cognitive enhancement) on 7-point scale ranging from very much improved (1) to very much worse (7). These two simple measures can be used in combination to identify the severity level of the patient's clinical status, whether that severity is too great to begin cognitive training, and to monitor changes in overall clinical status during the course of treatment.

10.6 Making Adjustments in Response to Assessment and Feedback

Collection of assessment data on cognitive and functional change is important for monitoring patient progress during cognitive enhancement. In order for such data to be useful during treatment it not only needs to be collected, but also it must be regularly reviewed, analyzed, and incorporated into treatment. Assessments taken prior to treatment are helpful in identifying areas of strength and challenge, determining the patient's predominant cognitive style, and tailoring the cognitive training program to the specific needs of the patient (see Chapter 9 for case examples). Data should also be collected throughout the course of treatment to monitor response and determine if any adjustments to the training program need to be made. It is recommended that at a minimum practitioners should collect cognitive and functional data prior to beginning cognitive enhancement, midway through cognitive training, and at the completion of treatment. Pre- and post-treatment assessments enable evaluation of the progress of the patient and efficacy of the training program. Mid-treatment assessments help the patient and practitioner take stock of progress made thus far during cognitive enhancement, and occur early enough to allow for adjustment during the program. The case of Anil provides an example of the utility of mid-treatment assessments of cognition in treatment planning and adjustment.

Case Study 10.1

Anil is a 40-year-old Indian American male who developed schizophrenia in his mid-20s. He has been stabilized on antipsychotic medication for over a decade, but struggles with maintaining work, planning his daily activities, and completing his household chores. He presents with a disorganized cognitive style, is difficult to follow during conversation, and his neuropsychological test results indicate that he has significant difficulty in planning and problem-solving (see Table 10.1). To address these issues, he and his clinician have begun cognitive enhancement using a top-down approach of executive function training with the PSSCogRehab suite. They have been utilizing the software in dedicated weekly 60-minute sessions for the past 3 months, and Anil's mid-treatment neuropsychological test results have just been completed (see Table 10.1). The clinician and Anil review his mid-treatment results and notice improvements in planning and problem-solving, but also have observed that during training, such progress has been slow and not of the magnitude that the clinician was expecting, given the amount of work Anil has put in to the training. They discuss the strengths of Anil's progress and also areas where Anil continues to struggle.

Anil reports that it is difficult to keep up with his co-workers on the assembly line, and that he is having trouble focusing his attention. He cannot make a decision or solve problems quickly because he is constantly distracted and is not able to sustain his attention beyond a few seconds at a time. The clinician notices that at baseline Anil did initially present with significant impairments in attention/vigilance, which appear to have continued from mid-treatment testing results (see Table 10.1). She suggests that the focus of training shift from executive function training to attention training, which she suspects will help address his challenges in sustained attention and also have downstream impact on his problem-solving and planning abilities. With Anil's permission, they switch from a top-down approach with PSSCogRehab to a bottom-up auditory training approach focused on improving attention using brainHQ. After several more months of cognitive enhancement, Anil becomes increasingly more organized, is able to maintain a conversation on the same topic for longer periods of time, and he is now able to keep up with most duties on his job. His end of treatment results indicate significant improvements in attention and processing speed, as well as additional marked gains in planning and problem-solving.

The scenario above describing Anil's progress through cognitive enhancement illustrates the importance of pre-treatment assessments of initial planning, and mid-treatment assessments for making important changes during the course of treatment. Anil noticed that he was improving by mid-treatment, but not enough to have a meaningful functional impact, and also noticed that his difficulties seemed to stem more from basic lower-order challenges in attention. This prompted his clinician to change the

Table 10.1 Pre-treatment, mid-treatment, and post-treatment neuropsychological test scores for Anil using the MATRICS Consensus Cognitive Battery

Domain	Pre-treatment Percentile (%)	Mid-treatment Percentile (%)	Post-treatment Percentile (%)
Speed of processing	20	20	50
Attention/vigilance	15	15	45
Working memory	55	50	55
Visual learning and memory	40	55	45
Verbal learning and memory	45	50	50
Reasoning and problem-solving	10	40	55
Social cognition	45	50	45

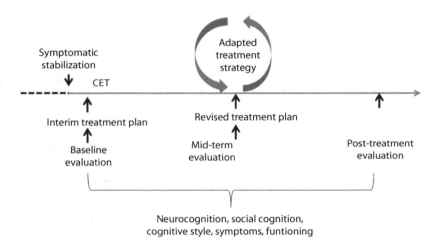

Figure 10.1 Adaptive strategy with cognitive enhancement based on pre-treatment and interim assessments

cognitive training program from a top-down to a bottom-up approach to see if improving Anil's attentional capacity could have a meaningful impact on his work and other life skill challenges. Of course, when the change occurred, neither Anil nor his clinician were certain of the outcome, but they used the best information available from Anil's pre- and mid-treatment assessments to collaboratively make a decision about the best use of Anil's time during cognitive training. In this case, that information was exceedingly helpful and implemented a more effective bottom-up approach to cognitive training for Anil, highlighting the importance of continuous assessment and monitoring of cognitive change throughout the treatment process.

Anil's case also illustrates the need to be flexible in the implementation of any cognitive enhancement program (see Figure 10.1). If the practitioner had continued to insist on using a higher-order training approach, gains made during treatment may have been more limited, as Anil's attentional challenges would not have been addressed. It is not unusual to learn information during the course of cognitive training that suggests a need for a change in the training approach or focus, especially when continuous assessment data are being collected over a meaningful, multi-month course of treatment. The practitioner should use such information to continually guide the treatment process, to determine when sufficient gains have been made to move to new cognitive domains, and to determine when to conclude treatment. Most evidence suggests that 60 hours of cognitive training are needed to achieve a meaningful cognitive response in patients with schizophrenia, but individual responses can vary remarkably, further underscoring the need to assess and monitor treatment progress for each individual patient.

10.7 Summary

- All cognitive enhancement programs should include standardized methods for assessing and monitoring patient response in terms of cognition and functioning.
- Clinical assessments are useful to include in cognitive enhancement programs to ensure that patients are stable enough to be eligible for inclusion and to determine whether cognitive change is due to treatment or other clinical factors.
- Interim assessments of patient progress provide an excellent opportunity to evaluate the effectiveness of the current training program and determine whether changes need to be made to support greater patient recovery.
- Nearly every important domain for assessment during cognitive enhancement has a validated, brief measure that is user-friendly and easy to implement in community practice.

Research in Cognitive Enhancement
Challenges and Opportunities

The field of cognitive enhancement interventions has made substantive progress over the past two decades, leading to considerable optimism. However, the results of studies generally show moderate effect sizes, and clearly, more rigorous basic and translational research is needed. Translational research applies discoveries from basic science (Bench-side, translational level T1) to enhance human health and well-being at the clinic level (translational level T2) and at the community level (translational level T3). Translational science is bidirectional, such that observations at the clinic and community levels can inform basic science research. It is important for the field to consider several critical methodological issues at each of these levels. We will address three levels of translational science to discuss the potential steps toward optimum development and implementation of cognitive enhancement interventions. We review promises and challenges facing the field in each of these research enterprises, and suggest potential directions for the future.

11.1 Translation from the Bench to the Humans (T1)

This level of translational research yields insights about human physiology and cognitive science for the development of novel interventions. Investigating animal models of schizophrenia and related disorders can be valuable in testing key predictions in cognitive enhancement research. For example, Lee (2012) examined whether cognitive training during adolescence can attenuate schizophrenia-like cognitive impairments in adulthood. They used rats with neonatal ventral hippocampus lesions, an established neurodevelopmental model of schizophrenia. Adolescent cognitive training prevented impairment in cognitive control and also enhanced cognition-associated synchrony of neural oscillations between the hippocampi, a measure of brain function that indexed cognitive ability. While such studies are promising, several challenges persist in T1 translational studies: animal models do not faithfully parallel the clinical syndromes or the complex cognitive impairments in human illnesses (Nestler & Hyman, 2010), and tests of cognition are only approximate analogs of the widely used human cognitive assessments, though considerable progress is being made (Pratt, 2012). The recent application of translational cognitive constructs for clinical research such as Cognitive Neuroscience Treatment Research to Improve Cognition in Schizophrenia (CNTRICS; see Chapter 1 for details) is a welcome step in this direction (Barch et al., 2009).

Animal models of complex psychiatric illnesses have been criticized for not having validity. An animal model ideally has to replicate the symptoms and signs of a human illness (face validity), have similar causes and mechanisms (construct validity), and must have similar outcomes with or without treatments (predictive validity; Keshavan,

Nasrallah, & Tandon, 2011; Keshavan et al., 2015). One well studied example of animal models is the impaired sensorimotor gating, as measured by Pre-Pulse Inhibition (PPI) of startle responses in rats. Imagine how an unexpected knock on your door will lead you to jump up with a startle response, but this startle can be reduced by first making a gentle knock on the door. PPI refers to the ability of such a non-startling "pre-pulse" to inhibit responding to the subsequent stimulus or "pulse" with a startle. Schizophrenia patients show PPI deficits, and PPI can easily be tested in rodents. Studies of mouse models using schizophrenia-associated genes have shown the usefulness of PPI models suggesting some face, predictive, and construct validity in schizophrenia studies (Powell, Weber, & Geyer, 2011).

However, such models have yet to yield novel therapeutic agents. A large part of this challenge lies in the substantive heterogeneity of schizophrenia. There is an increasing view that we may need to move beyond validity in our efforts to develop novel interventions. Swerdlow & Light (2016) have suggested that the field needs to move beyond simply a "find what's broke and fix it" approach; even an animal model that is not valid can have utility. Thus, it may be of value to identify aspects of spared neural function in schizophrenia patients, and investigate how such preserved neural mechanisms may be targeted by learning-based therapies in order to harness compensatory neuroplasticity (Swerdlow & Light, 2016). Extant animal models can potentially be repurposed to examine such questions.

11.2 Translation to Patients (T2)

The goal of this level of translational research is to investigate novel interventions in order to develop a basis for evidence-based practice. T2 translational studies seek to develop a knowledge base about the efficacy of therapeutic interventions in clinical settings. Several important issues need to be considered in designing studies of cognitive enhancement interventions (see Box 11.1).

Design Issues

A frequent consideration in designing studies of cognitive interventions is the decision of testing stand-alone treatments (e. g. [Fisher et al., 2009a, b] vs. integrated treatments such as CET [Eack et al., 2009; Hogarty et al., 2004] and IPT [Brenner et al., 1980]). While the latter approaches are likely to yield larger effect sizes and better generalization to real world outcomes, therapeutic mechanisms are harder to discern, and would require "dismantling" studies to elucidate the key ingredients of therapeutic effect. In recent years, NIMH has begun to support treatment studies which adopt an "experimental medicine" approach (Insel, 2015), in an effort to accelerate discovery and transfer of pharmacological treatments from bench to bedside. In this view, a clinical trial should identify a potential mechanism for the proposed treatment, to be used as a "proxy" target that the medication should be shown to "engage" (e.g. a receptor or enzyme), before moving to test effects on the desired clinical outcome. While this approach is promising for psychopharmacology, complex psychiatric illnesses such as schizophrenia with multifaceted, multiply determined symptoms pose substantive challenges to the project of identifying therapeutic targets for cognitive and behavioral interventions (Lewandowski et al., 2017) (see Figure 11.1).

Box 11.1 Points for consideration in the design, conduct, and review of cognitive enhancement intervention studies

Design considerations

Use of appropriate sample sizes
Randomization procedures
Blinding procedures
Operationalization and manualization of procedures
Measurement of fidelity to treatment approach
Considerations of predictors/moderators (e.g. concomitant medications, therapist engagement, adherence)

Study population

Use of appropriate intake criteria for study participants
Choice of appropriate controls
Reporting screen failures/retention/completion rates (consort diagrams)

Intervention considerations

Monotherapy or adjunct to another psychosocial treatment
Definition of control interventions
Drill and practice versus strategy training versus combination
Comprehensive versus targeted training
Targeting of social cognition

Outcome measures

Choice of appropriate cognitive and functional outcomes
A priori definition of primary, co-primary, and secondary outcomes
Cognitive measures (generalization of cognitive outcomes distinct from training tasks)
Functional outcomes (generalization to real-world function)
Measures at multiple levels of analysis (e.g. genes, molecules, cells, circuits, physiology, behavior, and self-report, as appropriate)

Analyses

Use of appropriate statistical tests
Controlling for confounding variables
Controlling for practice effects

Source: Adapted from Keshavan et al. (2014).

Choice of Control Groups

A control group is a group of participants who are not exposed to the intervention but are otherwise similar to an experimental group that receives a treatment under consideration. In choosing an appropriate control group, the investigator has to consider possible non-specific factors that may contribute to therapeutic benefits such as the length of the time spent in treatment, office setting, therapist factors, etc. Such non-specific factors are particularly likely in studies which utilize "Treatment as Usual" as the control group. An optimal approach is to use an active control intervention that matches the experimental group in regard to as many non-specific factors as possible, such as supportive therapy (Spaulding, 1992) or non-specific computer games (Fisher et al., 2009a). However, care should be taken to ensure that the "active control" intervention will not have the proposed

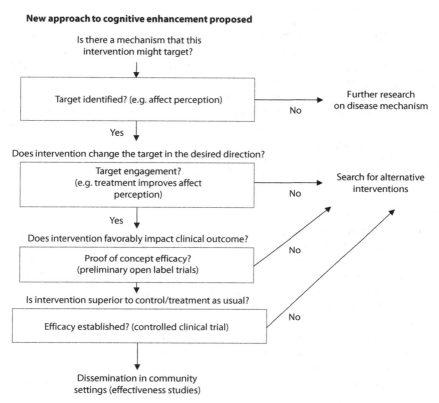

New approach to cognitive enhancement proposed

Is there a mechanism that this intervention might target?

Target identified? (e.g. affect perception)

No → Further research on disease mechanism

Yes ↓

Does intervention change the target in the desired direction?

Target engagement? (e.g. treatment improves affect perception)

No → Search for alternative interventions

Yes ↓

Does intervention favorably impact clinical outcome?

Proof of concept efficacy? (preliminary open label trials)

No

Is intervention superior to control/treatment as usual?

Efficacy established? (controlled clinical trial)

No

Dissemination in community settings (effectiveness studies)

Figure 11.1 The experimental medicine approach applied to development of cognitive enhancement interventions

therapeutic ingredient of the experimental intervention (e.g. cognitive training) so that we do not "throw out the baby with the bathwater."

Randomization

Investigators also need to consider differences in the characteristics of experimental and control groups in order to avoid the possible confounding effects of pre-existing group differences. Random assignment of participants to experimental and control interventions is therefore important, for ensuring that every participant is as likely to be placed in one group or the other. A simple way to do this is to flip a coin. It is also possible to generate random numbers using computer programs.

Blind Design

Another important problem in clinical trials is reporting bias. Participants may often cause bias by trying to please the investigator and therefore work harder to perform better or to feel better to meet the investigator's expectations. To address this problem, pharmacological studies typically blind the participants to the treatment by using placebos (which in Latin means "I shall please"). In psychotherapeutic research, placebo treatments are hard to design because of their nature being obvious to the participant. However, it may be possible to maintain blindness to treatment assignment by utilizing interventions that are similar to but do not contain the key therapeutic ingredient (e.g. cognitively non-demanding computer games), as discussed earlier.

Measurement Bias may also be introduced unknowingly by the assessors, by transmitting their own expectations to the participants. While this can be addressed in pharmacological studies by the research staff being blinded to the allocation status of subjects (drug versus placebo), it is not easy to accomplish for psychosocial treatments. One way to address this is to use centralized ratings of video assessments and to ensure that the outcomes are evaluated blind to subject allocation status.

Inference Testing

To investigate the possibility that differences observed between experimental and control groups may have occurred simply by chance, statistical testing is important. If the likelihood of an observed result is very low (e.g. conventionally less than 5%), the investigators may conclude that the results are due to the experimental intervention. However, it is to be kept in mind that if the sample size is large enough, even subtle differences may become statistically significant. It is therefore important to distinguish between statistical significance (which simply means that a change occurred because of treatment) and clinical significance (which means that the amount of improvement makes a meaningful difference for the patient). Clinical significance is expressed with effect sizes that are accompanied with confidence intervals rather than merely p values, and investigators should utilize both measures of uncertainty when evaluating their interventions.

Defining Populations

The efficacy of cognitive interventions is likely to be impacted by clinical diagnosis, age, baseline cognitive function, and the presence of limiting factors such as organic mental disorders, intellectual disability, and medications that affect cognitive function, such as anticholinergic medications. Because of the etiologic and phenotypic heterogeneity of psychotic disorders, it is unlikely that any particular neurocognitive deficit will be universal to all individuals within a diagnostic category. Different cognitive phenotypes may have a similar clinical presentation; not all individuals will demonstrate specific cognitive deficits of interest; and specific cognitive deficits may cut across disorders and healthy states (Hill et al., 2013). This raises the question of how to operationally define "case-ness" in selecting individuals for intervention studies. Thus, if the entry criteria consider only DSM or ICD diagnostic categories without addressing baseline neurocognitive heterogeneity, individuals for whom the proposed cognitive training intervention is not relevant could inadvertently be included in the sample.

Assessment of Moderators and Predictors

For prescriptive, personalized intervention strategies to be developed, one needs dense multi-modal baseline assessments of participants so that we can answer the question, "Who might best respond to which treatment?" In this manner, the feasibility of assessing putative moderators, as suggested by theory and research, could be explored in pilot studies. These putative moderators could then be examined in formal moderator analyses in subsequent studies with larger samples. Robust moderators thus identified could then be used as tailoring variables for more prescriptive treatment assignment (see Chapter 8 for a further discussion).

Neurobiological measures may provide additional predictors and moderators that may be more specific. For example, biomarkers derived from imaging, electrophysiology, or TMS might be used to assess neural reserve or plasticity. Genotype, reward sensitivity, motivational state, and internalized beliefs might also be valuable predictive factors. Keshavan et al. (2011) showed that baseline cortical thickness and surface area were predictive of earlier therapeutic response to Cognitive Enhancement Therapy. Genetic factors may also be relevant: Lindenmayer et al. (2015) recently showed that improvements with cognitive training in attention, verbal, and visual learning were predicted by baseline catechol O-methyl transferase (COMT) genotype data, favoring Met/Met and Val/Met over Val/Val groups.

The lack of comparability of cognitive measures across species has led to challenges in translation of cognitive enhancement approaches from animal models. The CNTRICS initiative seeks to harness cognitive neuroscience to develop a series of neuroscience-based assessments of cognition in schizophrenia (Moore et al., 2013); such approaches can be used in testing new cognitive interventions.

Defining Treatment Targets

Understanding the mechanisms driving behavioral change requires us to define the treatment target of the cognitive training intervention under study and to demonstrate target engagement. Primary or co-primary outcome measures (e.g. cognition, functioning) need to be explicitly identified at the outset, as should potential secondary outcomes of interest. Accordingly, preliminary proof of concept studies would seek to demonstrate that the intervention results in hypothesized changes in the hypothesized proximal target (e.g. a specific brain circuit, or a psychological process, such as working memory or attention bias). Larger studies would then formally interrogate mediational pathways and examine whether changes in the presumed target mediates or translates into clinical benefit. Care should be taken in distinguishing these two concepts (Baron & Kenny, 1986), as while mediation indicates the potential mechanisms by which an intervention works, moderation signifies for whom a treatment may be most beneficial.

We must also control for non-specific factors such as concomitant therapies that can influence behavioral outcomes unrelated to cognitive training. In schizophrenia (McGurk et al., 2007b), meta-analyses suggest that adjunctive psychosocial rehabilitation enhances cognitive training's impact on functional outcomes, but the specificity of this effect is unclear. Future studies need to quantify extra-protocol interventions, and assess outcomes to identify synergistic benefits and to develop optimized interventions.

Interpreting Meta-Analyses

Readers of treatment literature have to increasingly familiarize themselves with reviews and meta-analyses to get a big picture of emerging interventions. A meta-analysis is generated by the pooled statistical effects from different studies which may include large and small samples, those with versus without asymmetrical distributions, those with differing treatment delivery systems, and those with data collected from diverse settings. Even though most such analyses set criteria for study selection, such as randomization, blinding, and use of similar diagnostic criteria, the problem of "garbage in garbage out" has still to be guarded against. Often, the overall effect of meta-analyses is to give a higher weight to the smaller and more poorly designed studies and dilute the effects of larger and better designed studies (Hogarty, 2002). Meta-analyses, however, are justified in situations where there are a large number of well-designed studies that disagree and where the reader wants to identify an overall effect. The results of systematic reviews and meta-analyses also need to account for possible "file drawer effects" (i.e. studies whose negative results, despite their importance, may never have been published). One way to minimize file drawer effects is by including data from unpublished studies (the so-called "gray" literature), and to ensure that all clinical trials are pre-registered (see below). There are statistical ways of detecting publication bias, such as funnel plots (Flore & Wicherts, 2015). Another approach is mega-analysis in which the results of multiple studies (published and unpublished) are combined using individual-level data for a large number of patients, thereby increasing statistical power to detect differences in outcomes.

Clinical Trial Reforms

Recent studies have indicated that less than 50% of NIH-funded trials are published in peer-reviewed journals and about a third are not published at all. This means a lot of wasted taxpayer dollars! To address this problem, in recent years, NIH has begun an effort to streamline the clinical trial process and enhance its transparency. A clinical trial is defined by NIH as any intervention (which may or may not include placebo) to examine the effects on health-related biomedical or behavioral outcomes. This definition has been viewed as too broad by some scientists who have argued that studies addressing basic scientific questions (e.g. examining the effects of brain stimulation on cortical plasticity and not on clinical outcomes) may in this way be inappropriately classified as clinical trials. However, any intervention that could modify behavior and thereby have a health impact needs to carry a higher level of accountability, as expected for clinical trials. Since January 2017 NIMH has mandated that all clinical trials be registered on the website clinicaltrials.gov within 21 days after enrollment of the first participant, and that all results are posted on this website within 1 year of study completion. Increasingly, medical journals are requiring that clinical trials be publicly registered. To assist investigators, the NIH website now has many tools available online, such as hypothetical case studies, a decision tree, and a detailed section on Frequently Asked Questions (FAQ).

11.3 Translation from the Clinic to the Community: Dissemination and Implementation (T3)

A final and highly important consideration in translational research involves the dissemination of cognitive training into clinical and community practice. Many factors contribute to delays in the research-to-practice translation, including fundamental differences between efficacy studies and the usual care context. This research-to-practice "gap" has prompted calls to re-think the intervention development and testing process. Often the failure of translation stems from the interventions being developed in "ivory tower" university clinical settings, with tightly controlled designs and entry criteria, making generalization difficult. Medalia et al. (2017) have recently described the feasibility and acceptability of cognitive training in large-scale, geographically diverse, public-funded clinic settings in New York state. A reduction of referrals, enrollment, and utilization was seen when the program was extended from the development site to community settings. However, the majority (97%) of participants reported that cognitive remediation was either good, or excellent, suggesting high acceptability.

A "deployment-focused" model of intervention development and testing (Weisz et al., 2013), emphasizes incorporating information about typical patients, providers, settings and stakeholder perspectives (e.g. consumers, family members, providers, administrators, insurers, and payers) much earlier in the intervention testing process. Careful consideration of patient characteristics (e.g. common comorbidities), candidate interventions (e.g. scalability, complexity, patient burden, costs), potential providers (e.g. current competencies, training needs), and settings (e.g. capacity, competing demands, supervision infrastructure, reimbursement structure) will also likely facilitate the development of more practice-ready, scalable, cost-efficient interventions. Stakeholder support from payers and providers is also essential for successful implementation and sustainability of cognitive training programs.

Dissemination to Community Settings: Factors to Consider

Dissemination of cognitive training interventions into community settings is an important consideration (Keshavan et al., 2014). The efficacy–effectiveness gap results from many factors which contribute to delays in the research-to-practice translation (Tcheremissine et al., 2014).

Cost Considerations

Administrators and policymakers often balk at implementing evidence-based practices because of cost issues. It is important to keep in mind however that it is expensive to both not do the right things, and to not do things right! There is evidence that improving cognition is likely to enhance functional outcome and thereby reduce societal as well as personal costs of the illness. However, it is possible that additional costs will be incurred because of training and implementation which may not be easily covered through existing payment systems. There is recent evidence that cognitive treatments are cost-effective (Garrido et al., 2017; Yamaguchi, 2017). As the evidence base for cognitive training interventions is increasing, a critical barrier to implementation will be the development of payment models by which third-party insurers will reimburse for these types of interventions, which do not always resemble traditional individual and group therapies.

Effectiveness Considerations

Policymakers and other stakeholders frequently worry that services may not have an evidence base that supports implementation. There is increasing evidence for efficacy and generalizability of cognitive enhancement approaches and it is important for developers of these treatments to disseminate such evidence to key stakeholders. However, a greater number of effectiveness studies are clearly needed, as the majority of the evidence base in support of cognitive training interventions is derived from university-based clinical trials. Notable exceptions do exist, however, highlighting the feasibility and effectiveness of cognitive training for schizophrenia in more real-world settings (McGurk et al., 2007b) and samples (Eack et al., 2015).

Fidelity Issues

Effective implementation of therapeutic interventions in the community requires a high degree of standardization to ensure the needed precision for outcome evaluations. However, in routine community settings implementing such fidelity is challenging and may need to allow for frequent modifications to the original model (Aarons et al., 2011). Such modifications will inevitably lead to questions a given intervention has deviated significantly from the prescribed manual and whether such deviations lead to better or worse outcomes. Future implementation studies need to investigate how to adapt and develop practical guidelines and flexible fidelity metrics for evidence-based interventions in routine clinical settings and whether such adapted programs continue to lead to the desired clinical outcomes. The traditional approach in translating a clinic-based intervention to the community is to "develop-then-disseminate." This model may be cumbersome and inefficient; a knowledge translation approach such as that used by the Canadian Institutes of Health Research which integrates dissemination and implementation with knowledge acquisition in an action–knowledge cycle might be more effective (Srihari, Shah, & Keshavan, 2012).

Infrastructure and Funding Issues

Infrastructure components needed for cognitive enhancement approaches such as information systems and clinical record systems, etc. may not be uniformly available across diverse community settings. Frequent shifts in the leadership and staff as well as changing regulations and organizational structure could pose problems. Such problems are best addressed by ongoing dialog between those involved in treatment dissemination and those setting policy for overall infrastructure and funding.

Stages of Implementation

Implementation of cognitive enhancement interventions in community settings can take years. Frances Dark (Dark, 2016) has recently proposed a series of stages of such implementation, outlined in Figure 11.2. Successful implementation of evidence-based practices in community settings requires several steps. First, one needs to identify "*what*" is needed by the community, and is supported by evidence, Second, the question needs to be addressed of "*where*" implementation is to be carried out, and setting up, in a staged manner, the needed time and resources. The final task is "*how*" to ensure the necessary infrastructure by including key stakeholders such as providers, consumers, payers and policymakers, and program site teams; and using data to guide next steps and sustaining improvement (Metz & Albers, 2014). These steps will need to take an iterative approach, proceeding in successive cycles of planning, implementation, evaluation, and reflection (Figure 11.3).

Exploratory Phase

In this phase, the main goal is to build consensus among legislators, funders, and provider organizations related to implementation of cognitive enhancement approaches and also to address stakeholder concerns. Infrastructure readiness in terms of staffing information systems and training should also be explored. Approaches to measuring and monitoring fidelity and incorporating them into quality improvement mechanisms also need to be developed.

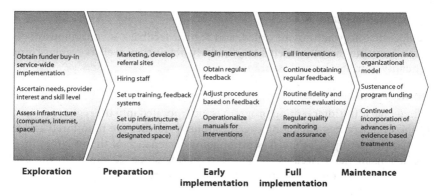

Figure 11.2 Dissemination of evidence-based practice (Dark, 2016)

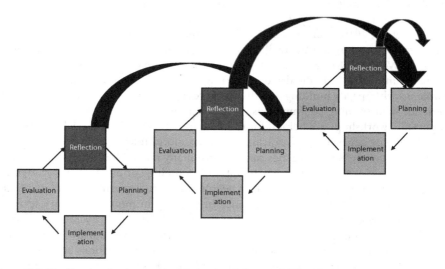

Figure 11.3 The Planning–Implementation–Evaluation–Reflection (PIER) cycle.

Preparatory Phase

The key goals in this phase are to identify and establish referral sites, develop marketing materials, and hiring staff. Steps should also be taken to train staff and set up infrastructure including computers, internet resources, and to identify designated space. Accessibility and transportation issues need to be examined and addressed. Feedback systems for optimal performance of cognitive training approach should also be set up.

Early Implementation Phase

In this phase the interventions are begun; regular feedback is obtained from participants as well as staff; such information is then used to iteratively improve intervention procedures. Operational manuals for the interventions are developed. Barriers to implementation are identified and addressed. Systems to manage data and efficient reporting are developed.

Full Implementation Phase

The therapeutic interventions are scaled, and regular feedback is continuously solicited. Fidelity and outcome measurements are regularly obtained as well as regular "program" audits, quality monitoring, and assurance.

Maintenance Phase

In this final phase, the intervention program is incorporated into the reguar services business of the organization. Changing organizational priorities are monitored and appropriate responses set up. Mechanisms for ongoing sustenance of the program including funding arrangements as well as collaborative partnerships. Advances in the evidence base for cognitive interventions are continuously explored and incorporated into intervention procedures.

Approaches to Training and Who to Train

Training workshops may by themselves not significantly impact practice patterns (Herschell et al., 2010; McHugh, 2010). Initial training programs followed by ongoing periodic case consulting, individually or in small groups may be effective (Schoenwald, Kelleher, & Weisz, 2008). While literature in this area of implementation science is scanty, it seems intuitive that individualized consulting and expert support gradually faded out in tandem with capacity building of individual providers will have the best results. In our experience with training community sites in Cognitive Enhancement Therapy, we find that periodic workshops are helpful for dividing the broad set of material to be learned and that ongoing supervision is critical to ensuring model fidelity.

Cognitive enhancement coaches can stem from any mental health discipline such as psychology, social work, nursing, rehabilitation, counseling, or psychiatry. Key prerequisites include experience in taking care of people with serious mental illness, familiarity with the psychosocial treatment, experience in working in multidisciplinary team settings, and a working knowledge of cognition and its deficits and psychotic illnesses. A master's degree in one of these disciplines is usually desired though not always mandatory. A cognitive enhancement trainer would have all of these qualifications and in addition have leadership experience, knowledge of the evidence base for cognitive enhancement approaches, and experience with training coaches and ongoing supervision.

The content of cognitive training interventions may be held both as immersion workshops as well as regular weekly or fortnightly supervision sessions. In such workshops one may include topics such as the nature and neurobiological basis of cognition and psychosis, the nature of brain plasticity and the theoretical models of cognitive enhancement approaches, methods for cognitive training and assessment, and the evidence-base for the efficacy of these interventions.

11.4 Digital Mental Health Applications for Cognitive Enhancement Approaches

The use of mobile phones and wearable devices in healthcare settings is steadily increasing in the general population, and even faster in the seriously mentally ill populations. They may offer a cost-effective way to deliver cognitive enhancement approaches. Smartphones may be able to reduce treatment time, and allow treatment delivery in the home without the need for expensive clinician involvement. Smartphones allow collection of passive (e.g. behavior and mobility via actigraphy and GPS data) and active behavior data (via survey data for symptom and cognitive function, as well as online cognitive tests), as well as the collection of physiological data (i.e. sleep, heart rate) using wearable devices such as Fitbit. Together, these data allow construction of a "digital phenotype" of each person that may be more reliable and sensitive for assessing day-to-day functioning than periodic clinical visits (Torous, Onnela, & Keshavan, 2017). The reliability and validity of a smartphone-based approach to assessing cognition has already been demonstrated (Sliwinski et al., 2016).

Use of mobile devices for cognitive interventions is only just beginning. A survey study showed a high degree of interest in brain training apps in the US, especially among the younger population (Torous et al., 2016). A recent paper reviewed four studies (involving 206 participants) comparing online interventions for memory and executive functioning in traumatic brain injury against a "placebo" (participants were given Internet resources on brain injury). No clear evidence of superiority was seen (Linden, 2016). A mobile cognitive training app has been developed for multiple sclerosis patients with cognitive impairments, and has been shown to be well-accepted and motivating, though efficacy has not yet been demonstrated (Tacchino et al., 2015). However, literature is sparse in this regard in smartphone-based cognitive interventions in schizophrenia or related disorders. The potential in this area is quite substantive, and more systematic work is needed to demonstrate efficacy, safety, and user engagement for these applications.

11.5 Emerging Treatment Targets for Cognitive Enhancement

As the field of cognitive training interventions is being established, and the efficacy of approaches on traditional neuropsychological targets of attention, memory, and problem-solving are being validated, new targets for intervention are also emerging as promising cognitive targets for improving functional recovery from schizophrenia and related conditions. Perhaps the most discussed and investigated novel target for cognitive training to date is the training of social cognition, or the ability to process and interpret socio-emotional information in oneself and others (Green et al., 2008; Newman, 2001). Social cognition training programs have emerged as an eclectic set of group- and computer-based approaches designed for enhancing such domains as theory of mind, perspective-taking, emotion perception and management, social cue recognition, and dysfunctional attributional styles (Kurtz & Richardson, 2011; see Chapters 5 and 6). Evidence to date suggests that the addition of social cognition training to traditional neurocognitive approaches to remediation confers significant benefits to ward functional outcomes (Mueller, Schmidt, & Roder, 2015), and some have hypothesized that this domain may be a critical link between neurocognitive challenges and functional disability in schizophrenia (Schmidt, 2011; Sergi et al., 2006). As such, social cognition represents one of the most promising new targets for remediation in schizophrenia and the field is working steadily to identify essential components to be addressed using cognitive training methods.

Metacognition is another fast-emerging treatment target. The ability to step back and recognize one's own personal cognitive strengths and challenges, as well as biases, is a key aspect of metacognitive processing that is impaired in schizophrenia (Moritz & Woodward, 2007) and may have functional consequences (Lysaker et al., 2010).

Delusion formation has long been thought to be, in part, the result of systematic cognitive biases, which metacognitive training seeks to correct. This approach is similar to cognitive behavioral therapy for psychosis (Kingdon & Turkington, 2005), but utilizes cognitive training approaches to identify and remediate key cognitive biases, such as jumping to conclusions and over-confidence in one's memory of events, through psychoeducation and the progressive practice of metacognitive exercises (Moritz et al., 2014). Metacognitive training also aims to improve general understanding of cognitive strengths and limitations, beyond biases, and helps participants to understand the impact of cognitive impairments on their daily lives and ways they may be able to limit the impact of these challenges.

Reward processing and motivation are two additional emerging therapeutic targets to which cognitive training interventions may be profitably directed. The hedonic and motivational challenges associated with schizophrenia, particularly among patients with the deficit syndrome (Kirkpatrick et al., 1989), are well-documented and largely untreated by antipsychotic medications or existing cognitive training programs (Carpenter & Buchanan, 2017). Further, motivation appears to be a critical factor to cognitive training outcomes, such as engagement and treatment efficacy (Saperstein & Medalia, 2015), and its direct targeting in treatment could significantly improve a variety of functional outcomes. To date, few studies have focused on the remediation of motivational deficits in schizophrenia using cognitive training approaches. However, traditional motivational interviewing methods can enhance treatment adherence to cognitive training programs (Fiszdon et al., 2015). Others have focused more directly on reward processing, aiming at developing leisure activities, and hobbies in patients to enhance their motivation and hedonic processing (Velligan et al., 2015). To date, however, studies have not been conducted using cognitive training methods to enhance motivation through computerized routines, and development of such approaches to target this important domain is an essential direction for future research.

11.6 Summary

- While cognitive enhancement approaches are effective, many questions remain, and systematic research is of high priority.
- Research in cognitive training needs to proceed in all three levels of translational research: bench to human studies, to clinical settings, and from clinical settings to the community.
- Clinical studies of cognitive enhancement need to consider specific issues in design, measurement, analysis, and interpretation.
- Community-wide dissemination and implementation require "buy in" from policymakers, mental health administrators, and other stakeholders, careful planning, implementation, and iterative fidelity, and outcome evaluations and improvements to be sustainable.
- Emerging and promising targets for cognitive remediation include social cognition, metacognition, motivation and reward processing. Treatment delivery in community settings using digital, mobile technology is a promising development.

Glossary

Amygdala. A brain region, located in the medial temporal lobe, known to mediate emotion processing

Anosognosia. A known neurological condition with impaired awareness of one's own neurological disability such as stroke

Attributional style. The way in which one makes sense of social events in life

Brain Computer Interface (BCI). Approaches that involve enabling control of computers and other assistive devices by using signals from the brain

Brief Assessment of Cognition in Schizophrenia (BACS). Brief, performance-based battery for neurocognitive assessment in schizophrenia

brainHQ. Bottom-up, computer-based neurocognitive training program focused on auditory processing

Cingulate cortex. A brain region, located in the medial frontal lobe, known to mediate selective attention, error monitoring, and executive function

Cognitive Enhancement. A set of approaches, ranging from pharmacological to psychosocial, to improve attention, memory, problem-solving, social understanding, and/or other aspects of cognition in neuropsychiatric conditions. Synonymous with cognitive training, cognitive remediation, and cognitive rehabilitation, but less stigmatizing and more widely applicable to non-disordered populations

Cognitive Enhancement Therapy. A specific approach to cognitive enhancement for schizophrenia originally developed by Hogarty and colleagues. See Hogarty and Greenwald (2006), www.CognitiveEnhancementTherapy.com for more details.

Cognitive flexibility. A neurocognitive process that supports the shifting of behavior across contexts and enables the identification and use of alternative problem-solving strategies

Cognitive Style. Clustered profiles of cognitive challenges used as a heuristic for reducing heterogeneity in patient presentation and for guiding cognitive enhancement

Cognitive Styles and Social Cognition Eligibility Interview. Interview-based assessment of social and non-social cognitive challenges originally designed for identifying significant cognitive impairments indicative of a need for treatment in Cognitive Enhancement Therapy

Cognitive Training. See Cognitive Enhancement

Cognitive Rehabilitation. See Cognitive Enhancement

Cognitive Remediation. See Cognitive Enhancement

Cognitive Remediation and Functional Adaptation Skills Training. An integrated computerized cognitive remediation with group-based behavioral skills training for schizophrenia developed by Bowie and colleagues

CogPack. Suite of computer-based neurocognitive training programs focused on attention, memory, and problem-solving developed by Marker Software

Context appraisal. A person's ability to judge social cues from information in the social context, and awareness of the roles, rules, and goals that characterize different, sometimes ambiguous social situations

Cognitive Neuroscience Treatment Research in Schizophrenia (CNTRICS). A battery of tests based on cognitive neuroscience constructs that may have better neural validity and may be translatable to experimental animal models

Continuous Performance Test (CPT). A test of sustained attention where a series of stimuli are presented, and the individual has to respond each time a target stimulus appears, e.g. whenever an X appears after an A

Critical windows. Learning and neuroplasticity are thought to occur within finite windows, early "critical periods." Adaptive or maladaptive experiences or insults to the developing brain during these critical periods can have lasting behavioral consequences

Dementia praecox. A term originally introduced by Benedict Morel for a chronic psychotic illness and further described by Emil Kraepelin and delineated from manic depressive illness. Dementia Praecox was later termed schizophrenia by Eugen Bleuler.

Dorsolateral prefrontal cortex. A brain region, located in the frontal lobe, known to mediate working memory and executive function

Emotion Perception. Social-cognitive ability

involving the accurate recognition and understanding of emotions in others, usually with regard to the face or vocal prosody

Epigenetics. Study of heritable changes in gene expression that occur without changes in the DNA sequence

Event-related potential (ERP). A brain response resulting from a specific sensory, cognitive, or motor event. ERPs are used to evaluate brain function, and are measured using electroencephalogram (EEG).

Executive function. Activities such as problem-solving, planning, and shifting between two or more tasks

Experience-dependent neuroplasticity. Very early in development, experience and its resulting neuronal activity can shape neuronal response properties irrespective of an organism's attention to a stimulus.

Explicit memory. A type of memory that involves a conscious sense of remembering and recall of autobiographical or factual information

Foresight. The ability to think of the long-term consequences of one's behavior and use this information to guide present and future actions

Fusiform gyrus. A brain region, located in the medial temporal lobe, known to mediate face processing

Growth mindset. The concept, developed by Carol Dweck, in which one's intellectual capability is not fixed but to a large extent is under one's own control

Hebbian learning. When two neurons repeatedly or persistently fire together, some change takes place in one or both cells such that the efficiency of neuronal activity is increased. The adage "neurons that fire together wire together" stems from this view first proposed by Donald O. Hebb.

Hippocampus. A brain region, located in the medial temporal lobe, known to mediate memory and spatial navigation

Implicit memory. A type of memory that does not involve a conscious sense of recall; an example of the latter is the person not consciously recalling the steps of how to ride a bicycle but being able to do so when needed.

Insight. A multidimensional concept that includes accurate self-awareness, correct attribution, and recognition of one's own illness and need for treatment

Integrated Psychological Therapy (IPT). An integrated, group-based neurocognitive and social-cognitive training model for schizophrenia developed by Brenner and colleagues

Long-term Potentiation (LTP). A phenomenon whereby repeated signal transmission from one neuron leads to long-lasting enhancement of the action potential (the activity of the nerve cell when it fires) transmission in the signal in the receiving neuron. LTP is the basis of neuroplasticity.

Measurement and Treatment Research to Improve Cognition in Schizophrenia (MATRICS). A battery of tests which has been developed in recent years for assessment of cognition in schizophrenia.

MATRICS Consensus Cognitive Battery (MCCB). The gold standard for cognitive assessments for clinical trial studies and assesses seven domains of cognitive functions using ten tests

Metacognition. It has been defined as "thinking about thinking". This includes self-monitoring, regulation as well as knowledge of ones' own mental operations.

Micro Expressions Training Tools. Computer-based social cognition training program focused on improving facial emotion perception and understanding developed by Paul Ekman

Mayer-Salovey-Caruso Emotional Intelligence Test (MSCEIT). A performance-based measure of emotional intelligence covering the domains of emotion perception, facilitation, understanding, and management

n-back task. A test of working memory. In the n-back test, a sequence of stimuli are presented, and subject has to indicate when the new stimulus (e.g. a number or letter) matches the one from n stimuli earlier in the sequence. n can be adjusted to vary the difficulty level of the task.

Neuropsychological Educational Approach to Remediation (NEAR). An eclectic and flexible group-based approach to neurocognitive training for schizophrenia developed by Medalia and colleagues

Neurocognition. A composite term used to refer to non-social cognitive processes involving attention, memory, and executive function, commonly assessed with standardized intelligence or neuropsychological tests

Neuromodulation. A variety of approaches to stimulate or inhibit brain functions by external devices

Orientation Remedial Module (ORM). Computer-based cognitive training program focused on attention developed by Ben-Yishay and colleagues

Penn Computerized Neurocognitive Battery. Computerized neurocognitive assessment suite that can be used to monitor cognitive enhancement outcomes

Perspective taking. The ability to take viewpoints of other people (*mentalizing or theory of mind*) and make inferences about their mental states based on available social context information

Posit Science. Creators of the auditory neurocognitive training program, brainHQ, led by Michael Merzenich

Plasticity. The property of the brain to change (be molded, or sculpted) by experience

PSSCogRehab. Suite of computer-based neurocognitive training programs focused on improving attention, memory, and problem-solving developed by Odie Bracy

Psychoeducation. The provision of education surrounding mental health generally, and cognitive strengths and challenges, specifically, with regard to cognitive enhancement

Scaffolding. A concept used in cognitive enhancement approaches, is derived from scaffolds which support a building's development, and serves as a framework for a learner to perform within the limits of his/her capacity.

Schizophrenia Cognition Rating Scales (SCORS). A brief, interview-based assessment of neurocognitive and social-cognitive for schizophrenia

Specific Levels of Functioning Scale (SLOF). A commonly used measure of functional outcome assessed by collateral informants, such as family members and clinicians

Social cognition. A composite term used to refer to the cognitive processes involved in the understanding, interpretation, and management of socio-emotional information in oneself and others

Social Cognition and Interaction Training (SCIT). A group-based social cognition training program for patients with schizophrenia developed by Penn, Roberts, and colleagues

Social Cognitive Skills Training. A group-based approach to social cognition training for schizophrenia developed by William Horan and colleagues

Social context appraisal. The ability to understand the rules and norms of behavior in changing, diverse, and spontaneous social situations

Social cue recognition. Social-cognitive ability involving the accurate perception of non-verbal signals presented by others, including facial expressions, body posture, and tone of voice

Social perception. General term for social-cognitive abilities involving the accurate perception of social context, expressions of emotion, and other non-verbal social cues. Includes social context appraisal, emotion perception, and social cue recognition, among other social-cognitive abilities.

Spindle sleep. An interesting type of oscillations during non-rapid eye movement (NREM) called sleep spindles are thought to play a role in synaptic changes and sleep-dependent memory consolidation

Stroop test. This is a test of selective attention. In this task, the subject is asked to name the colors of the words and not read the words, as fast as he/she can. Thus, if the word "BLUE" is printed in red (i.e. incongruant words), the subject should say "RED". Naming the color of the word takes longer and causes more errors when the color of the ink does not match the name of the color.

Supported employment. An important concept in vocational rehabilitation in which a "place and train" approach is used in contrast to the traditional model where the person is trained first and then placed in an occupational setting.

The Awareness of Social Inferences Test (TASIT). This test assesses mentalizing (perspective taking, or theory of mind) processes depicted in videotaped interactions between adults, such as forming inferences about others' intentions and detecting white lies and sarcasm.

Theory of mind. See Perspective taking

Therapeutic alliance. The relationship between a clinician and patient which can be an important factor that determines outcome with treatment

Thinking Skills for Work. An integrated computerized cognitive remediation and individualized supported employment program for patients with schizophrenia developed by Susan McGurk and colleagues

Transcranial direct current stimulation (tDCS). It uses direct currents to shift the resting membrane potentials of underlying neurons.

Transcranial magnetic stimulation (TMS). It uses focal magnetic fields to stimulate the brain. The resultant electric currents then depolarize the underlying cortex, thus inducing action potentials in targeted brain regions. It has been used to study in vivo cortical plasticity in schizophrenia.

UPSA. A widely used performance-based measure of functional capacity, the UCSD Performance-based Skills Assessment (UPSA) was developed by Thomas Patterson and colleagues

WHOQOL-BREF. A widely used, brief assessment of quality of life developed by the World Health Organization and useful for monitoring changes in functional outcome and quality of life

Working memory. A specific form of short-term memory used to hold limited information in the mind to perform a task

References

Aarons, G. A., Hurlburt, M., & Horwitz, S. M. (2011). Advancing a conceptual model of evidence-based practice implementation in public service sectors. *Administration and Policy in Mental Health*, *38*(1), 4–23.

Adcock, R. A., Dale, C., Fisher, M. et al. (2009). When top-down meets bottom-up: auditory training enhances verbal memory in schizophrenia. *Schizophrenia Bulletin*, *35*(6), 1132–1141.

Adler, A. A. (1927). *Practice and Theory of Individual Psychology*. New York, NY: Harcourt, Brace & Co.

Adolphs, R., Gosselin, F., Buchanan, T. W. et al. (2005). A mechanism for impaired fear recognition after amygdala damage. *Nature*, *433*(7021), 68–72.

Allison, T., Puce, A., & McCarthy, G. (2000). Social perception from visual cues: role of the STS region. *Trends in Cognitive Sciences*, *4*(7), 267–278.

Amador, X. (2010). *I Am Not Sick, I Don't Need Help! How to Help Someone with Mental Illness Accept Treatment* (10th Anniversary edn.). New York, NY: Vida Press.

Amador, X. F., Strauss, D. H., Yale, S. A. et al. (1993). Assessment of insight in psychosis. *American Journal of Psychiatry*, *150*, 873–879.

Anaya, C., Martinez Aran, A., Ayuso-Mateos, J. L. et al. (2012). A systematic review of cognitive remediation for schizo-affective and affective disorders. *Journal of Affective Disorders*, *142*(1–3), 13–21. doi: 10.1016/j.jad.2012.04.020

Anderson, C., Reiss, D., & Hogarty, G. W. (1986). *Schizophrenia and the Family: A Practitioner's Guide to Psychoeducation and Management*. Guilford Press, May 12, 1986

Andrade, K. C., Spoormaker, V. I., Dresler, M. et al. (2011). Sleep spindles and hippocampal functional connectivity in human NREM sleep. *Journal of Neuroscience*, *31*(28), 10331–10339. doi: 10.1523/JNEUROSCI.5660-10.2011

Andreasen, N. C. (1983). *Scale for the Assessment of Negative Symptoms*. Iowa City, IA: University of Iowa Press. (1984). *Scale for the Assessment of Positive Symptoms*. Iowa City, IA: University of Iowa Press.

Andreasen, N. C., Flaum, M., Swayze, V. W., Tyrrell, G., & Arndt, S. (1990). Positive and negative symptoms in schizophrenia: a critical reappraisal. *Archives of General Psychiatry*, *47*(7), 615–621.

Army Individual Test Battery. (1944). *PsycTESTS Dataset*. Washington, DC: American Psychological Association (APA).

American Psychiatric Association. (2013). *Diagnostic and Statistical Manual of Mental Disorders (DSM-5®)* (5th edn.). Washington, DC: American Psychiatric Association.

Atkins, A. S., Tseng, T., Vaughan, A. et al. (2017). Validation of the tablet-administered Brief Assessment of Cognition (BAC App). *Schizophrenia Research*, *181*, 100–106. doi: 10.1016/j.schres.2016.10.010

Autry, A. E., & Monteggia, L. M. (2012). Brain-derived neurotrophic factor and neuropsychiatric disorders. *Pharmacological Reviews*, *64*(2), 238–258. doi: 10.1124/pr.111.005108

Baddeley, A., & Wilson, B. A. (1994). When implicit learning fails: amnesia and the problem of error elimination. *Neuropsychologia*, *32*(1), 53–68.

Banks, S. J., Eddy, K. T., Angstadt, M., Nathan, P. J., & Phan, K. L. (2007). Amygdala–frontal connectivity during emotion regulation. *Social Cognitive and Affective Neuroscience*, *2*(4), 303–312.

Barch, D. M., & Carter, C. S. (2005). Amphetamine improves cognitive function in medicated individuals with schizophrenia and in healthy volunteers. *Schizophrenia Research*, *77*, 43–58.

Barch, D. M., Berman, M. G., Engle, R. et al. (2009). CNTRICS final task selection: working memory. *Schizophrenia Bulletin*, *35*, 136–152.

Baron, R. M., & Kenny, D. A. (1986). The moderator–mediator variable distinction in social psychological research: conceptual, strategic, and statistical considerations. *Journal of Personality and Social Psychology, 51*(6), 1173–1182.

Baron-Cohen S., Wheelwright S., Hill J., Raste Y., & Plumb I. (2001). The "Reading the Mind in the Eyes" Test revised version: a study with normal adults, and adults with Asperger syndrome or high-functioning autism. *Journal of Child Psychology and Psychiatry, 42*(2), 241–51.

Bell, M., Bryson, G., Greig, T., Corcoran, C., & Wexler, B. E. (2001). Neurocognitive enhancement therapy with work therapy. *Archives of General Psychiatry, 58*(8), 763. doi: 10.1001/archpsyc.58.8.763

Bell, M., Bryson, G., & Wexler, B. E. (2003). Cognitive remediation of working memory deficits: durability of training effects in severely impaired and less severely impaired schizophrenia. *Acta Psychiatrica Scandinavica, 108*(2), 101–109.

Ben-Yishay, Y., Piasetsky, E. B., & Rattok, J. (1985). A Systematic Method for Ameliorating Disorders in Basic Attention. In A. L. B. M. J. Meir, & L. Diller (Eds.), *Neuropsychological Rehabilitation* (pp. 165–181). New York, NY: Guilford Press.

Ben-Yishay, Y., & Prigatano, G. P. (1990). Cognitive Remediation. In: M. Rosenthal, M. R. Bond, E. R. Griffith, & J. D. Miller (Eds.), *Rehabilitation of the adult and child with traumatic brain injury* (pp. 393–409). Philadelphia, PA: F A Davis.

Benoit, A., Harvey, P. O., Bherer, L., & Lepage, M. (2016). Does the beck cognitive insight scale predict response to cognitive remediation in Schizophrenia? *Schizophrenia Research and Treatment,* 2016, 6371856. doi: 10.1155/2016/6371856. Epub 2016 Jul 19.

Berman, K. F. (1987). Cortical "stress tests" in schizophrenia: regional cerebral blood flow studies. *Biological Psychiatry, 22*(11), 1304–1326.

Birchwood, M., Spencer, E., & McGovern, D. (2000). Schizophrenia: early warning signs. *Advances in Psychiatric Treatment, 6*(2), 93–101.

Bitanihirwe, B. K., & Woo, T. U. (2014). Perineuronal nets and schizophrenia: the importance of neuronal coatings. *Neuroscience & Biobehavioral Reviews, 45C,* 85–99. doi: 10.1016/j.neubiorev.2014.03.018

Bond, G. R., & Drake, R. E. (2014). Making the case for IPS supported employment. *Administration and Policy in Mental Health and Mental Health Services Research, 41*(1), 69–73.

Bora, E., & Murray, R. M. (2013). Meta-analysis of cognitive deficits in ultra-high risk to psychosis and first-episode psychosis: do the cognitive deficits progress over, or after, the onset of psychosis? *Schizophrenia Bulletin, 40*(4), 744–755. doi: 10.1093/schbul/sbt085

Bordon, N., O'Rourke, S., & Hutton, P. (2017). The feasibility and clinical benefits of improving facial affect recognition impairments in schizophrenia: systematic review and meta-analysis. *Schizophrenia Research, 188,* 3–12. doi: 10.1016/j.schres .2017.01.014

Boroojerdi, B. P. M., Kopylev, L., Wharton, C. M., Cohen, L. G., & Grafman, J. (2001). Enhancing analogic reasoning with rTMS over the left prefrontal cortex. *Neurology,* 56, 526–528.

Bosia, M., Bechi, M., Marino, E. et al. (2007). Influence of Catechol-O-Methyltransferase Val158Met polymorphism on neuropsychological and functional outcomes of classical rehabilitation and cognitive remediation in schizophrenia. *Neuroscience Letters, 417*(3), 271–274. doi: 10.1016/j.neulet.2007.02.076

Bosia, M., Zanoletti, A., Spangaro, M. et al. (2014). Factors affecting cognitive remediation response in schizophrenia: the role of COMT gene and antipsychotic treatment. *Psychiatry Research, 217*(1–2), 9–14. doi: 10.1016/j.psychres.2014.02.015

Bowie, C. R., Grossman, M., Gupta, M., Oyewumi, L. K., & Harvey, P. D. (2013). Cognitive remediation in schizophrenia: efficacy and effectiveness in patients with early versus long-term course of illness. *Early Intervention in Psychiatry, 8*(1), 32–38. doi: 10.1111/eip.12029

Bowie, C. R., McGurk, S. R., Mausbach, B., Patterson, T. L., & Harvey, P. D. (2012). Combined cognitive remediation and functional skills training for schizophrenia: effects on cognition, functional competence, and real-world behavior. *American Journal of Psychiatry, 169*(7), 710–718. doi: 10.1176/appi.ajp .2012.11091337

Bozikas, V. P., Kosmidis, M. H., Kioperlidou, K., & Karavatos, A. (2004). Relationship between psychopathology and cognitive functioning in schizophrenia. *Comprehensive Psychiatry*, *45*(5), 392–400.

Bracy, O. L. (1994). *PSSCogRehab*. Indianapolis, IN: Psychological Software Services Inc.

Brady, R. O. J., Tandon, N., Masters, G. A. et al. (2017). Differential brain network activity across mood states in bipolar disorder. *Journal Affective Disorders*, *207*, 367–376.

Breitborde, N. J. K., Woolverton, C., Dawson, S. C. et al. (2015). Meta-cognitive skills training enhances computerized cognitive remediation outcomes among individuals with first-episode psychosis. *Early Intervention in Psychiatry*, *11*(3), 244–249. doi: 10.1111/eip.12289

Brenner, H., Stramke, W., Mewes, J., Liese, F., & Seeger, G. (1980). A treatment program, based on training of cognitive and communicative functions, in the rehabilitation of chronic schizophrenic patients (author's translation). *Der Nervenarzt*, *51*(2), 106–112.

Brenner, H. D. (2000). Psychological therapy in schizophrenia: what is the evidence? *Acta Psychiatrica Scandinavica*, *102*(s407), 74–77. doi: 10.1034/j.1600-0447.2000.00014.x

Brenner, H. D., Roder, V., Hodel, B. et al. (1994). *Integrated Psychological Therapy for Schizophrenic Patients (IPT)*. Seattle, WA: Hogrefe & Huber Publishers.

Broadbent, D. (1958). *Perception and Communication*. London: Pergamon Press.

Brothers, L., Ring, B., & Kling, A. (1990). Response of neurons in the macaque amygdala to complex social stimuli. *Behavioural Brain Research*, *41*(3), 199–213.

Brown, P. C., Roediger, H. L., & Mcdaniel, M. A. (2017). *Make It Stick: The Science of Successful Learning*. Cambridge, MA: Harvard University Press.

Brown, R. P., Gerbarg, P. L., & Muench, F. (2013). Breathing practices for treatment of psychiatric and stress-related medical conditions. *Psychiatric Clinics of North America*, *36*(1), 121–140.

Browning, M., Holmes, E. A., & Harmer, C. J. (2010). The modification of attentional bias to emotional information: A review of the techniques, mechanisms, and relevance to emotional disorders. *Cognitive Affective & Behavioral Neuroscience*, *10*(1), 8–20.

Buchanan, R. W., & Carpenter, W. T. (1994). Domains of psychopathology: an approach to the reduction of heterogeneity in schizophrenia. *Journal of Nervous and Mental Disease*, *182*(4), 193–204.

Buchanan, R. W., Keefe, R. S. E., Lieberman, J. A. et al. (2011). A randomized clinical trial of MK-0777 for the treatment of cognitive impairments in people with schizophrenia. *Biological Psychiatry*, *69*(5), 442–449.

Buonomano, D. V., & Merzenich, M. M. (1998). Cortical plasticity: from synapses to maps. *Annual Review of Neuroscience*, *21*, 149–186.

Cannon, T. D., Chung, Y., He, G. et al. (2015). Progressive reduction in cortical thickness as psychosis develops: a multisite longitudinal neuroimaging study of youth at elevated clinical risk. *Biological Psychiatry*, *77*(2), 147–157.

Cappa, S. F., Sandrini, M., Rossini, P. M., Sosta, K., & Miniussi, C. (2002). The role of the left frontal lobe in action naming: rTMS evidence. *Neurology*, *59*(10), 720–723.

Carelli, L., Solca, F., Faini, A. et al. (2017). Brain–computer interface for clinical purposes: cognitive assessment and rehabilitation. *BioMed Research International*, 2017:1695290. doi: 10.1155/2017/1695290. Epub 2017.

Carpenter Jr., W. T., & Buchanan, R. W. (2017). Negative symptom therapeutics. *Schizophrenia Bulletin*, *43*(4), 681–682.

Carpenter, S. K., & Mueller, F. E. (2013). The effects of interleaving versus blocking on foreign language pronunciation learning. *Memory & Cognition*, *41*(5), 671–682.

Carter, C. S., & Barch, D. M. (2007). Cognitive neuroscience-based approaches to measuring and improving treatment effects on cognition in schizophrenia: the CNTRICS initiative. *Schizophrenia Bulletin*, *33*(5), 1131–1137.

Carter, C. S., Botvinick, M. M., Cohen, J. D. (1999). The contribution of the anterior cingulate cortex to executive processes in cognition. *Reviews in the Neurosciences*, *10*(1), 49–57.

Carter, C. S., Robertson, L. C., Nordahl, T. E. (1992). Abnormal processing of irrelevant information in chronic schizophrenia: selective enhancement of Stroop facilitation. *Psychiatry Research*, *41*(2), 137–146.

Cavus, I., Reinhart, R. M., Roach, B. J. et al. (2012). Impaired visual cortical plasticity in schizophrenia. *Biological Psychiatry, 71*(6), 512–520. doi: 10.1016/j.biopsych .2012.01.013

Cella, M., & Wykes, T. (2017). The nuts and bolts of cognitive remediation: exploring how different training components relate to cognitive and functional gains. *Schizophrenia Research*, 2017 Sep 14. pii: S0920-9964(17)30571-6. doi: 10.1016/j .schres.2017.09.012. [Epub ahead of print]. PMID: 28919130.

Cella, M., Reeder, C., & Wykes, T. (2015). Cognitive remediation in schizophrenia – now it is really getting personal. *Current Opinion in Behavioral Sciences, 4*, 147–151.

Cepeda, N. J., Pashler, H., Vul, E., Wixted, J. T., & Rohrer, D. (2006). Distributed practice in verbal recall tasks: a review and quantitative synthesis. *Psychological Bulletin, 132*, 354–380.

Choi, J., & Medalia, A. (2010). Intrinsic motivation and learning in a schizophrenia spectrum sample. *Schizophrenia Research, 118*(1–3), 12–19. doi: 10.1016/j.schres .2009.08.001

(2005). Factors associated with a positive response to cognitive remediation in a community psychiatric sample. *Psychiatric Services, 56*(5), 602–604. doi: 10.1176/appi .ps.56.5.602

Chua, S., Wright, I., Poline, J. et al. (1997). Grey matter correlates of syndromes in schizophrenia. A semi-automated analysis of structural magnetic resonance images. *British Journal of Psychiatry, 170*(5), 406–410.

Clapp, W. C., Kirk, I. J., Hamm, J. P., Shepherd, D., & Teyler, T. J. (2005). Induction of LTP in the human auditory cortex by sensory stimulation. *European Journal of Neuroscience, 22*(5), 1135–1140. doi: 10.1111/j.1460-9568.2005.04293.x

Clapp, W. C., Zaehle, T., Lutz, K. et al. (2005). Effects of long-term potentiation in the human visual cortex: a functional magnetic resonance imaging study. *NeuroReport, 16*(18), 1977–1980.

Claro, S., Paunesku, D., & Dweck, C. S. (2016). Growth mindset tempers the effects of poverty on academic achievement. *Proceedings of the National Academy of Sciences of the United States of America, 113*(31), 8664–8668.

Clementz, B. A., Sweeney, J. A., Hamm, J. P. et al. (2016). Identification of distinct psychosis biotypes using brain-based biomarkers. *American Journal of Psychiatry, 173*(4), 373–384. doi: 10.1176/appi .ajp.2015.14091200

Combs, D. R., Adams, S. D., Penn, D. L., Roberts, D., Tiegreen, J., & Stem, P. (2007). Social Cognition and Interaction Training (SCIT) for inpatients with schizophrenia spectrum disorders: Preliminary findings. *Schizophrenia Research, 91*(1), 112–116.

Cooper, G., & Sweller, J. (1987). Effects of schema acquisition and rule automation on mathematical problem-solving transfer. *Journal of Educational Psychology, 79*(4), 347–362.

Corcoran, R., Mercer, G., & Frith, C. D. (1995). Schizophrenia symptomatology and social inference: investigating "theory of mind" in people with schizophrenia. *Schizophrenia Research 17*, 5–13.

Corrigan, P. W., & Green, M. F. (1993). Schizophrenic patients' sensitivity to social cues: the role of abstraction. *American Journal of Psychiatry, 150*(4), 589–594.

Couture, S. M., Penn, D. L., & Roberts, D. L. (2006). The functional significance of social cognition in schizophrenia. *Schizophrenia Bulletin, 32* (supplement 1), S44–S63.

Dark, F. (2016). Implementation and Dissemination of Evidence-Based Mental Health Practices. In A. Medalia, & C. R. Bowie (Eds.), *Cognitive Remediation to Improve Functional Outcomes* (pp. 117–137). New York, NY: Oxford University Press.

Daskalakis, Z. J., Christensen, B. K., Fitzgerald, P. B., & Chen, R. (2008). Dysfunctional neural plasticity in patients with schizophrenia. *Archives of General Psychiatry, 65*(4), 378–385. doi: 10.1001/ archpsyc.65.4.378

Davis, M. C., Green, M. F., Lee, J. et al. (2014). Oxytocin-augmented social cognitive skills training in schizophrenia. *Neuropsychopharmacology, 39*(9), 2070–2077. doi: 10.1038/npp.2014.68

De Vignemont, F., & Singer, T. (2006). The empathic brain: how, when and why? *Trends in Cognitive Sciences, 10*(10), 435–441.

Deci, E. L., & Ryan, R. M. (1987). The support of autonomy and the control of behavior. *Journal of Personality and Social Psychology, 53*(6), 1024–1037.

Deegan, P. E., & Drake, R. E. (2006). Shared decision making and medication management in the recovery process. *Psychiatric Services, 57*(11), 1636–1639.

Demirtas-Tatlidede, A., Vahabzadeh-Hagh, A. M., & Pascual-Leone, A. (2013). Can noninvasive brain stimulation enhance cognition in neuropsychiatric disorders? *Neuropharmacology, 64*, 566–578.

Deutsch, S. I., Schwartz, B. L., Schooler, N. R. et al. (2013). Targeting alpha-7 nicotinic neurotransmission in schizophrenia: a novel agonist strategy. *Schizophrenia Research, 148*(1–3), 138–144.

Diagnostic and Statistical Manual of Mental Disorders. (2000). *Text Revision (DSM-IV-TR)* (4th edn). Arlington, VA: American Psychiatric Association.

Dickinson, D., Ragland, J. D., Gold, J. M., & Gur, R. C. (2008). General and specific cognitive deficits in schizophrenia: Goliath defeats David? *Biological Psychiatry, 64*(9), 823–827. doi: 10.1016/j.biopsych .2008.04.005

Dixon, R. A., & Bäckman, L. (1992–1993). The concept of compensation in cognitive aging: the case of prose processing in adulthood. *International Journal of Aging and Human Development, 36*(3), 199–217.

Dixon, R. A., et al. (2008). *Cognitive Rehabilitation.* Cambridge, UK: Cambridge University Press.

Dutra, L., Stathopoulou, G., Basden, S. L. et al. (2008). A meta-analytic review of psychosocial interventions for substance use disorders. *American Journal of Psychiatry, 165*(2), 179–187. doi: 10.1176/appi.ajp .2007.06111851

Dweck, C. S. (2015). Growth. *British Journal of Educational Psychology, 85*(2), 242–245. doi: 10.1111/bjep.12072

Eack, S., Greenwald, D., Hogarty, S. et al. (2009). Cognitive enhancement therapy for early-course schizophrenia: effects of a two-year randomized controlled trial. *Psychiatric Services, 60*(11). doi: 10.1176/appi.ps.60.11.1468

Eack, S. M. (2012). Cognitive remediation: a new generation of psychosocial interventions for people with schizophrenia. *Social Work, 57*(3), 235–246. doi: 10.1093/ sw/sws008

(2013). Cognitive Enhancement Therapy. In D. L. Roberts & D. L. Penn (Eds.), *Social Cognition in Schizophrenia* (pp. 335–357). New York, NY: Oxford University Press.

Eack, S. M., Greeno, C. G., Pogue-Geile, M. F. et al. (2010). Assessing social-cognitive deficits in schizophrenia with the Mayer-Salovey-Caruso Emotional Intelligence Test. *Schizophrenia Bulletin, 36*(2), 370–380.

Eack, S. M., Greenwald, D. P., Hogarty, S. S. et al. (2009). Cognitive enhancement therapy for early-course schizophrenia: effects of a two-year randomized controlled trial. *Psychiatric Services, 60*(11), 1468–1476. doi: 10.1176/appi.ps.60.11.1468

Eack, S. M., Greenwald, D. P., Hogarty, S. S., & Keshavan, M. S. (2010). One-year durability of the effects of cognitive enhancement therapy on functional outcome in early schizophrenia. *Schizophrenia Research, 120*(1–3), 210–216. doi: 10.1016/j.schres .2010.03.042

Eack, S. M., Hogarty, G. E., Cho, R. Y. et al. (2010). Neuroprotective effects of cognitive enhancement therapy against gray matter loss in early schizophrenia: results from a 2-year randomized controlled trial. *Archives of General Psychiatry, 67*(7), 674–682. doi: 10.1001/ archgenpsychiatry.2010.63

Eack, S. M., Hogarty, G. E., Greenwald, D. P., Hogarty, S. S., & Keshavan, M. S. (2007). Cognitive enhancement therapy improves emotional intelligence in early course schizophrenia: preliminary effects. *Schizophrenia Research, 89*(1–3), 308–311. doi: 10.1016/j.schres .2006.08.018

Eack, S. M., Hogarty, S. S., Bangalore, S. S., Keshavan, M. S., & Cornelius, J. R. (2016). Patterns of substance use during cognitive enhancement therapy: an 18-month randomized feasibility study. *Journal of Dual Diagnosis, 12*(1), 74–82. doi: 10.1080/15504263.2016.1145778

Eack, S. M., Hogarty, S. S., Greenwald, D. P. et al. (2015). Cognitive enhancement therapy in substance misusing schizophrenia: results of an 18-month feasibility trial. *Schizophrenia Research, 161*(2–3), 478–483. doi: 10.1016/j.schres.2014.11.017

(2017). Cognitive enhancement therapy for adult autism spectrum disorder: results of an 18-month randomized clinical trial. *Autism Research, 11*(3), 519–530. doi: 10.1002/aur.1913

Eack, S. M., Hogarty, G. E., Cho, R. Y. et al. (2010). Neuroprotective effects of cognitive enhancement therapy against gray matter loss in early schizophrenia: results from a 2-year randomized controlled trial. *Archives of General Psychiatry, 67*(7), 674–682.

Eack, S. M., & Keshavan, M. S. (2008). Foresight in schizophrenia: a potentially unique and relevant factor to functional disability. *Psychiatric Services, 59*(3), 256–260. doi: 10.1176/ps.2008.59.3.256

Eack, S. M., Mesholam-Gately, R. I., Greenwald, D. P., Hogarty, S. S., & Keshavan, M. S. (2013). Negative symptom improvement during cognitive rehabilitation: results from a 2-year trial of cognitive enhancement therapy. *Psychiatry Research, 209*(1), 21–26. doi: 10.1016/j .psychres.2013.03.020

Ehrenreich, H., Degner, D., Meller, J. et al. (2004). Erythropoietin: a candidate compound for neuroprotection in schizophrenia. *Molecular Psychiatry, 9*(1), 42–54.

Eisch, A. J., Cameron, H. A., Encinas, J. M. et al. (2008). Adult neurogenesis, mental health, and mental illness: hope or hype? *Journal of Neuroscience 28*(46), 11785–11791. doi: 10.1523/ JNEUROSCI.3798-08.2008

Ekman, P. (2004). *Micro Expressions Training Tools*. Retrieved from www.paulekman .com/micro-expressions-training-tools. Accessed November 8, 2018.

Elbert, T., Pantev, C., Wienbruch. C., Rockstroh, B., & Taub, E. (1995). Increased cortical representation of the fingers of the left hand in string players. *Science, 270*(5234), 305–307.

Emerson, R. W. (2000). *Compensation*. New York, NY: Caldwell.

Erickson, M. A., Ruffle, A., & Gold, J. M. (2016). A meta-analysis of mismatch negativity in schizophrenia: from clinical risk to disease specificity and progression. *Biological Psychiatry, 79*(12), 980–987. doi: 10.1016/j.biopsych.2015.08.025

Farrow, T. F., Hunter, M. D., Haque, R., & Spence, S. A. (2006). Modafinil and unconstrained motor activity in schizophrenia: double-blind crossover placebo-controlled trial. *British Journal of Psychiatry, 189*, 461–462.

Faustman, W. O., & Overall, J. E. (1999). Brief Psychiatric Rating Scale. In M. Maruish (Ed.), *The Use of Psychological Testing for Treatment Planning and Outcome Assessment* (2nd edn., pp. 791–830). Hillsdale, NJ: Erlbaum.

Feinberg, I. (1982–1983). Schizophrenia: caused by a fault in programmed synaptic elimination during adolescence? *Journal of Psychiatric Research, 17*(4), 319–334.

Fenton, W. S. (1997). We can talk: individual psychotherapy for schizophrenia. *American Journal of Psychiatry, 154*(11), 1493–1495. doi: 10.1176/ajp.154.11.1493

Fett, A. K., Viechtbauer, W., Dominguez, M. D. et al. (2011). The relationship between neurocognition and social cognition with functional outcomes in schizophrenia: a meta-analysis. *Neuroscience & Biobehavioral Reviews, 35*(3), 573–588. doi: 10.1016/j .neubiorev.2010.07.001

Fisher, E., Achilles, S., & Tonnies, H. (2014). Predictive genetic testing, risk communication, and risk perception: an international expert meeting in Berlin, Germany. *Journal of Community Genetics, 5*(1), 1–5. doi: 10.1007/ s12687-013-0177-6

Fisher, M., Holland, C., Merzenich, M. M., & Vinogradov, S. (2009a). Using neuroplasticity-based auditory training to improve verbal memory in schizophrenia. *American Journal of Psychiatry, 166*(7), 805–811. doi: 10.1176/appi.ajp.2009 .08050757

Fisher, M., Holland, C., Subramaniam, K., & Vinogradov, S. (2009b). Neuroplasticity-based cognitive training in schizophrenia: an interim report on the effects 6 months later. *Schizophrenia Bulletin, 36*(4), 869–879. doi: 10.1093/schbul/sbn170

Fisher, M., Loewy, R., Carter, C. et al. (2015). Neuroplasticity-based auditory training via laptop computer improves cognition in young individuals with recent onset schizophrenia. *Schizophrenia Bulletin, 41*(1), 250–258.

Fiszdon, J. M., Kurtz, M. M., Choi, J., Bell, M. D., & Martino, S. (2015). Motivational interviewing to increase cognitive rehabilitation adherence in schizophrenia. *Schizophrenia Bulletin*, *42*(2), 327–334.

Fitzgerald, P. B., Brown, T. L., Marston, N. A. et al. (2004). Reduced plastic brain responses in schizophrenia: a transcranial magnetic stimulation study. *Schizophrenia Research*, *71*(1), 17–26. doi: 10.1016/j.schres .2004.01.018

Flavell, J. H. (1979). Metacognition and cognitive monitoring: a new area of cognitive–developmental inquiry. *American Psychologist*, *34*(10), 906–911.

Flore, P. C., & Wicherts, J. M. (2015). Does stereotype threat influence performance of girls in stereotyped domains? A meta-analysis. *Journal of School Psychology*, *53*(1), 25–44.

Fogel, S., Martin, N., Lafortune, M. et al. (2012). NREM sleep oscillations and brain plasticity in aging. *Frontiers in Neurology*, *3*, 1–7. doi: 10.3389/ fneur.2012.00176

Frank, A. F., & Gunderson, J. G. (1990). The role of the therapeutic alliance in the treatment of schizophrenia. Relationship to course and outcome. *Archives of General Psychiatry*, *47*(1), 228–236.

Frantseva, M. V., Fitzgerald, P. B., Chen, R. et al. (2008). Evidence for impaired long-term potentiation in schizophrenia and its relationship to motor skill learning. *Cerebral Cortex*, *18*(5), 990–996. doi: 10.1093/cercor/ bhm151

Fredrick, M. M., Mintz, J., Roberts, D. L. et al. (2015). Is cognitive adaptation training (CAT) compensatory, restorative, or both? *Schizophrenia Research*, *166*(1), 290–296. doi: 10.1016/j.schres.2015.06.003

Frommann, N., Streit, M., & Wölwer, W. (2003). Remediation of facial affect recognition impairments in patients with schizophrenia: a new training program. *Psychiatry Research*, *117*(3), 281–284. doi: 10.1016/ s0165-1781(03)00039-8

Fujiwara, H., Yassin, W., & Murai, T. (2015). Neuroimaging studies of social cognition in schizophrenia. *Psychiatry and Clinical Neurosciences*, *69*(5), 259–267.

Gallego, J. A., Robinson, D. G., Sevy, S. M. et al. (2011). Time to treatment response in first episode schizophrenia: should acute treatment trials last several months? *Journal of Clinical Psychiatry*, *72*(12), 1691.

Garety, P., Joyce, E., Jolley, S. et al. (2013). Neuropsychological functioning and jumping to conclusions in delusions. *Schizophrenia Research*, *150*(2), 570–574. doi: 10.1016/j.schres.2013.08.035

Garrido, G., Penadés, R., Barrios, M. et al. (2017). Computer-assisted cognitive remediation therapy in schizophrenia: durability of the effects and cost-utility analysis. *Psychiatry Research*, *254*, 198–204.

Gioia, G., Isquith, P. K., Guy, S. C., Kenworthy, L. (2000). Reviewed by Baron, I.S. "Test Review: Behavior Rating Inventory of Executive Function". *Child Neuropsychology*. *6*(3), 235–238.

Giuliano, A. J., Li, H., Mesholam-Gately, R. I. et al. (2012). Neurocognition in the psychosis risk syndrome: a quantitative and qualitative review. *Current Pharmaceutical Design*, *18*(4), 399–415.

Glantz, L. A., & Lewis, D. A. (2000). Decreased dendritic spine density on prefrontal cortical pyramidal neurons in schizophrenia. *Archives of General Psychiatry*, *57*(1), 65–73.

Gold, J. M., Hahn, B., Strauss, G. P., & Waltz, J. A. (2009). Turning it upside down: areas of preserved cognitive function in schizophrenia. *Neuropsychology Review*, *19*(3), 294–311.

Goldberg, T. E., Keefe, R. S., Goldman, R. S., Robinson, D. G., & Harvey, P. D. (2010). Circumstances under which practice does not make perfect: a review of the practice effect literature in schizophrenia and its relevance to clinical treatment studies. *Neuropsychopharmacology*, *35*(5), 1053–1062.

Goldberg, T. E., Ragland, J. D., Torrey, E. F. et al. (1990). Neuropsychological assessment of monozygotic twins discordant for schizophrenia. *Archives of General Psychiatry*, *47*(11), 1066–1072.

Goldman-Rakic, P. S. (1994). Working memory dysfunction in schizophrenia. *Journal of Neuropsychiatry and Clinical Neurosciences*, *6*(4), 348–357.

Goldman-Rakic, P. S., & Selemon, L. D. (1997). Functional and anatomical aspects of prefrontal pathology in schizophrenia. *Schizophrenia Bulletin*, *23*(3), 437–458.

Gonzalez, R., Pacheco-Colón, I., Duperrouzel, J. C., & Hawes, S. W. (2017). Does cannabis use cause declines in neuropsychological functioning? A review of longitudinal studies. *Journal of the International Neuropsychological Society*, *23*(9–10), 893–902.

Green, M. F. (2000). Neurocognitive deficits and functional outcome in schizophrenia: are we measuring the "right stuff"? *Schizophrenia Bulletin*, *26*, 119–136.

Green, M. F., Nuechterlein, K. H., Gold, J. M. et al. (2004). Approaching a consensus cognitive battery for clinical trials in schizophrenia: the NIMH-MATRICS conference to select cognitive domains and test criteria. *Biological Psychiatry*, *56*(5), 301–307. doi: 10.1016/j.biopsych .2004.06.023

Green, M. F., Penn, D. L., Bentall, R. et al. (2008). Social cognition in schizophrenia: an NIMH workshop on definitions, assessment, and research opportunities. *Schizophrenia Bulletin*, *34*(6), 1211–1220.

Greeno, J. G. (1989). On the Nature of Competence: Principles for Understanding in a Domain©. In L. B. Resnick (Ed.), *Knowing, Learning, and Instruction: Essays in Honor of Robert Glaser* (pp. 125–186). Hillsdale, NJ: Erlbaum.

Greenwood, K., Hung, C. F., Tropeano, M., McGuffin, P., & Wykes, T. (2011). No association between the Catechol-O-Methyltransferase (COMT) Val158Met polymorphism and cognitive improvement following cognitive remediation therapy (CRT) in schizophrenia. *Neuroscience Letters*, *496*(2), 65–69.

Gur, R. C., Ragland, J. D., Moberg, P. J. et al. (2001). Computerized neurocognitive scanning: I. methodology and validation in healthy people. *Neuropsychopharmacology*, *25*(5), 766–776.

Gur, R. C., Richard, J., Hughett, P. et al. (2010). A cognitive neuroscience-based computerized battery for efficient measurement of individual differences: standardization and initial construct validation. *Journal of Neuroscience Methods*, *187*(2), 254–262. doi: 10.1016/j.jneumeth .2009.11.017

Guy, W. (1976). *ECDEU Assessment for Psychopharmacology* (Revised edn.). Rockville, MD: National Institute of Mental Health.

Hamann, J., Mendel, R., Cohen, R. et al. (2009). Psychiatrists' use of shared decision making in the treatment of schizophrenia: patient characteristics and decision topics. *Psychiatric Services*, *60*(8), 1107–1112.

Hamann, S. B., Ely, T. D., Hoffman, J. M., & Kilts, C. D. (2002). Ecstasy and agony: activation of the human amygdala in positive and negative emotion. *Psychological Science*, *13*(2), 135–141.

Harrow, M., Jobe, T. H., & Faull, R. N. (2012). Do all schizophrenia patients need antipsychotic treatment continuously throughout their lifetime? A 20-year longitudinal study. *Psychological Medicine*, *42*(10), 2145–2155.

Harvey, P. D., Raykov, T., Twamley, E. W. et al. (2011). Validating the measurement of real-world functional outcomes: phase I results of the VALERO study. *American Journal of Psychiatry*, *168*(11), 1195–1201. doi: 10.1176/appi.ajp.2011.10121723

Hasan, A., Nitsche, M. A., Herrmann, M. et al. (2012). Impaired long-term depression in schizophrenia: a cathodal tDCS pilot study. *Brain Stimulation*, *5*(4), 475–483. doi: 10.1016/j.brs.2011.08.004

Haut, K. M., Lim, K. O., & MacDonald, A., 3rd. (2010). Prefrontal cortical changes following cognitive training in patients with chronic schizophrenia: effects of practice, generalization, and specificity. *Neuropsychopharmacology*, *35*(9), 1850–1859. doi: 10.1038/npp.2010.52

Heaton, R. K. (1980). *A Manual for the Wisconsin Card Sorting Test*. Odessa, FL: Psychological Assessment Resources Inc.

Heaton, R. K., Chelune, G. J., Talley, J. L., Kay, G. G., & Curtiss, G. (1993). *Wisconsin Card Sorting Test Manual: Revised and Expanded*. Odessa, FL: Psychological Assessment Resources Inc.

Hebb, D. O. (1949). *Organization of Behavior: A Neuropsychological Theory*. New York, NY: John Wiley.

Heinrichs, R. W., & Zakzanis, K. K. (1998). Neurocognitive deficit in schizophrenia: a quantitative review of the evidence. *Neuropsychology*, *12*(3), 426.

Hemsley, D. (1977). What have cognitive deficits to do with schizophrenic symptoms? *British Journal of Psychiatry, 130*(2), 167–173.

Herbener, E. S., Hill, S. K., Marvin, R. W., & Sweeney, J. A. (2005). Effects of antipsychotic treatment on emotion perception deficits in first-episode schizophrenia. *American Journal of Psychiatry, 162*(9), 1746–1748. doi: 10.1176/appi.ajp.162.9.1746

Herschell, A. D., Kolko, D. J., Baumann, B. L., & Davis, A. C. (2010). The role of therapist training in the implementation of psychosocial treatments: a review and critique with recommendations. *Clinical Psychology Review, 30*, 448–466.

Hill, S. K., Reilly, J. L., Keefe, R. S., et al. (2013). Neuropsychological impairments in schizophrenia and psychotic bipolar disorder: findings from the Bipolar-Schizophrenia Network on Intermediate Phenotypes (B-SNIP) study. *American Journal of Psychiatry, 170*(11), 1275–1284.

Hogarty, G. E. (1974). Drug and sociotherapy in the aftercare of schizophrenic patients. *Archives of General Psychiatry, 31*(5), 609. doi: 10.1001/archpsyc.1974.01760170011002

(2002). *Personal Therapy for Schizophrenia and Related Disorders.* New York, NY: Guilford Press.

Hogarty, G. E., & Flesher, S. (1999). Practice principles of cognitive enhancement therapy for schizophrenia. *Schizophrenia Bulletin, 25*(4), 693–708.

Hogarty, G. E., & Greenwald, D. P. (2006). *Cognitive Enhancement Therapy: The Training Manual.* Pittsburgh, PA: CET Training, LLC.

Hogarty, G. E., Goldberg, S. C., Schooler, N. R., & the Collaborative Study Group. (1974). Drug and sociotherapy in the aftercare of schizophrenic patients: III. Adjustment of nonrelapsed patients. *Archives of General Psychiatry, 31*(5), 609–618.

Hogarty, G. E., Flesher, S., Ulrich, R. et al. (2004). Cognitive enhancement therapy for schizophrenia: effects of a 2-year randomized trial on cognition and behavior. *Archives of General Psychiatry, 61*(9), 866–876. doi: 10.1001/archpsyc.61.9.866

Hogarty, G. E., & Greenwald, D. P. (2006). Cognitive Enhancement Therapy. www.cognitiveenhancementtherapy.com/manual/. Accessed November 8, 2018.

Hooker, C. I., Bruce, L., Fisher, M. et al. (2012). Neural activity during emotion recognition after combined cognitive plus social cognitive training in schizophrenia. *Schizophrenia Research, 139*(1–3), 53–59. doi: 10.1016/j.schres.2012.05.009

Hooker, C. I., Carol, E. E., Eisenstein, T. J. et al. (2014). A pilot study of cognitive training in clinical high risk for psychosis: initial evidence of cognitive benefit. *Schizophrenia Research, 157*(1–3), 314–316. doi: 10.1016/j.schres.2014.05.034

Horan, W. P., Kern, R. S., Shokat-Fadai, K. et al. (2009). Social cognitive skills training in schizophrenia: an initial efficacy study of stabilized outpatients. *Schizophrenia Research, 107*(1), 47–54. doi: 10.1016/j.schres.2008.09.006

Horan, W. P., Kern, R. S., Tripp, C. et al. (2011). Efficacy and specificity of social cognitive skills training for outpatients with psychotic disorders. *Journal of Psychiatric Research, 45*(8), 1113–1122. doi: 10.1016/j.jpsychires.2011.01.015

Hubel, D. H., & Wiesel, T. N. (1959). Receptive fields of single neurones in the cat's striate cortex. *Journal of Physiology, 148*, 574–591.

Huddy, V., Reeder, C., Kontis, D., Wykes, T., & Stahl, D. (2012). The effect of working alliance on adherence and outcome in cognitive remediation therapy. *Journal of Nervous and Mental Disease, 200*(7), 614–619.

Hunter, M. D., Ganesan, V., Wilkinson, I. D., & Spence, S. A. (2006). Impact of modafinil on prefrontal executive function in schizophrenia. *American Journal of Psychiatry, 163*, 2184–2186.

Huttenlocher, P. R. (1979). Synaptic density in human frontal cortex-developmental changes and effects of aging. *Brain Research, 163*(2), 195–205.

Insel, T., Cuthbert, B., Garvey, M. et al. (2010). Research Domain Criteria (RDoC): toward a new classification framework for research on mental disorders. *American Journal of Psychiatry, 167*(7), 748–751. doi: 10.1176/appi.ajp.2010.09091379

Insel, T. R. (2015). The NIMH experimental medicine initiative. *World Psychiatry, 14*(2), 151–153.

James, W. (1890). *Principles of Psychology* (Vol. 2). Mineola, NY: Dover Publications.

Jarskog, L. F., Lowy, M. T., Grove, R. A. et al. (2015). A Phase II study of a histamine H 3 receptor antagonist GSK239512 for cognitive impairment in stable schizophrenia subjects on antipsychotic therapy. *Schizophrenia Research, 164*(1), 136–142.

Javitt, D. C. (2009). When doors of perception close: bottom-up models of disrupted cognition in schizophrenia. *Annual Review of Clinical Psychology, 5*(1), 249–275. doi: 10.1146/annurev.clinpsy.032408.153502

Javitt, D. C., Shelley, A. M., & Ritter, W. (2000). Associated deficits in mismatch negativity generation and tone matching in schizophrenia. *Clinical Neurophysiology, 111*(10), 1733–1737. doi: 10.1016/ s1388-2457(00)00377-1

Kabat-Zinn, J. (1996). *Full Catastrophe Living: How to Cope with Stress, Pain and Illness Using Mindfulness Meditation.* London, UK: Piatkus.

Kane, J. M., Robinson, D. G., Schooler, N. R. et al. (2015). Comprehensive versus usual community care for first-episode psychosis: 2-year outcomes from the NIMH RAISE early treatment program. *American Journal of Psychiatry, 173*(4), 362–372.

Kanwisher, N., McDermott, J., & Chun, M. M. (1997). The fusiform face area: a module in human extrastriate cortex specialized for face perception. *Journal of Neuroscience, 17*(11), 4302–4311.

Karson, C., Duffy, R. A., Eramo, A., Nylander, A. G., & Offord, S. J. (2016). Long-term outcomes of antipsychotic treatment in patients with first-episode schizophrenia: a systematic review. *Neuropsychiatric Disease and Treatment, 6*(12), 57–67.

Keech, B., Crowe, S., & Hocking, D. R. (2018). Intranasal oxytocin, social cognition and neurodevelopmental disorders: a meta-analysis. *Psychoneuroendocrinology, 87*, 9–19.

Keefe, R. (2004). The brief assessment of cognition in schizophrenia: reliability, sensitivity, and comparison with a standard neurocognitive battery. *Schizophrenia Research, 68*(2–3), 283–297. doi: 10.1016/j .schres.2003.09.011

Keefe, R. S., Bilder, R. M., Davis, S. M. et al. (2007). Neurocognitive effects of antipsychotic medications in patients with chronic schizophrenia in the CATIE Trial. *Archives of General Psychiatry, 64*(6), 633–647.

Keefe, R. S., Eesley, C. E., & Poe, M. P. (2005). Defining a cognitive function decrement in schizophrenia. *Biological Psychiatry, 57*(6), 688–691.

Keefe, R. S., Poe, M., Walker, T. M., Kang, J. W., & Harvey, P. D. (2006). The schizophrenia cognition rating scale: an interview-based assessment and its relationship to cognition, real-world functioning, and functional capacity. *American Journal of Psychiatry, 163*(3), 426–432. doi: 10.1176/appi.ajp.163.3.426

Keefe, R. S., Silva, S. G., Perkins, D. O., & Lieberman, J. A. (1999). The effects of atypical antipsychotic drugs on neurocognitive impairment in schizophrenia: a review and meta-analysis. *Schizophrenia Bulletin, 25*(2), 201–222.

Keefe, R. S. E. (2007). Neurocognitive effects of antipsychotic medications in patients with chronic schizophrenia in the CATIE Trial. *Archives of General Psychiatry, 64*(6), 633–647. doi: 10.1001/archpsyc.64.6.633

Keefe, R. S. E., Poe, M., Walker, T. M., Kang, J. W., & Harvey, P. D. (2006). The schizophrenia cognition rating scale: an interview-based assessment and its relationship to cognition, real-world functioning, and functional capacity. *American Journal of Psychiatry, 163*(3), 426–432. doi: 10.1176/appi.ajp.163.3.426

Keefe, R. S. E., Vinogradov, S., Medalia, A. et al. (2012). Feasibility and pilot efficacy results from the multisite Cognitive Remediation in the Schizophrenia Trials Network (CRSTN) randomized controlled trial. *Journal of Clinical Psychiatry, 73*(07), 1016–1022. doi: 10.4088/jcp.11m07100 (2010). Report from the working group conference on multisite trial design for cognitive remediation in schizophrenia. *Schizophrenia Bulletin, 37*(5), 1057–1065. doi: 10.1093/schbul/sbq010

Kern, R. S., Wallace, C. J., Hellman, S. G., Womack, L. M., & Green, M. F. (1996). A training procedure for remediating WCST deficits in chronic psychotic patients: An adaptation of errorless learning principles. *Journal of Psychiatric Research, 30*(4), 283–294.

Kerns, J. G., Cohen, J. D., MacDonald, A. W., 3rd et al. (2005). Decreased conflict- and error-related activity in the anterior cingulate cortex in subjects with schizophrenia. *American Journal of Psychiatry, 162*(10), 1833–1839. doi: 10.1176/appi.ajp.162.10.1833

Keshavan, M., Kulkarni, S., Bhojraj, T. et al. (2010). Premorbid cognitive deficits in young relatives of schizophrenia patients. *Frontiers in Human Neuroscience*, 3(62). doi: 10.3389/neuro.09.062.2009

Keshavan, M. S. (1999). Development, disease and degeneration in schizophrenia: a unitary pathophysiological model. *Journal of Psychiatric Research*, 33(6), 513–521.

Keshavan, M. S., & Eack, S. (2014). Psychosocial Treatments for Chronic Psychosis. In G. O. Gabbard (Ed.), *Gabbard's Treatments of Psychiatric Disorders* (5th edn., pp. 197–212). Washington, DC: American Psychiatric Publishing.

Keshavan, M. S., Anderson, S., & Pettegrew, J. W. (1994). Is schizophrenia due to excessive synaptic pruning in the prefrontal cortex? The Feinberg hypothesis revisited. *Journal of Psychiatric Research*, 28(3), 239–265.

Keshavan, M. S., Eack, S. M., Prasad, K. M., Haller, C. S., & Cho, R. Y. (2017). Longitudinal functional brain imaging study in early course schizophrenia before and after cognitive enhancement therapy. *NeuroImage*, 151, 55–64. doi: 10.1016/j.neuroimage.2016.11.060

Keshavan, M. S., Eack, S. M., Wojtalik, J. A., et al. (2011). A broad cortical reserve accelerates response to cognitive enhancement therapy in early course schizophrenia. *Schizophrenia Research*, 130(1–3), 123–129. doi: 10.1016/j.schres.2011.05.001

Keshavan, M. S., Giedd, J., Lau, J. Y. F., Lewis, D. A., & Paus, T. (2014). Changes in the adolescent brain and the pathophysiology of psychotic disorders. *Lancet Psychiatry*, 1(7), 549–558. doi: 10.1016/S2215-0366(14)00081-9

Keshavan, M. S., & Hogarty, G. E. (1999). Brain maturational processes and delayed onset in schizophrenia. *Development and Psychopathology*, 11(3), 525–543. doi: 10.1017/s0954579499002199

Keshavan, M. S., Lawler, A. N., Nasrallah, H. A., & Tandon, R. (2017). New drug developments in psychosis: challenges, opportunities and strategies. *Progress in Neurobiology*, 152, 3–20.

Keshavan, M. S., Mehta, U. M., Padmanabhan, J. L., & Shah, J. L. (2015). Dysplasticity, metaplasticity, and schizophrenia: implications for risk, illness, and novel interventions. *Development and Psychopathology*, 27(2), 615–635.

Keshavan, M. S., Nasrallah, H. A., & Tandon, R. (2011). Schizophrenia, "Just the Facts" 6. Moving ahead with the schizophrenia concept: from the elephant to the mouse. *Schizophrenia Research*, 127(1), 3–13.

Keshavan, M. S., Rabinowitz, J., DeSmedt, G., Harvey, P. D., & Schooler, N. (2004). Correlates of insight in first episode psychosis. *Schizophrenia Research*, 70(2), 187–194.

Keshavan, M. S., Vinogradov, S., Rumsey, J., Sherrill, J., & Wagner, A. (2014). Cognitive training in mental disorders: update and future directions. *American Journal of Psychiatry*, 171(5), 510–522. doi: 10.1176/appi.ajp.2013.13081075

Kingdon, D. G., & Turkington, D. (1994). *Cognitive-Behavioral Therapy of Schizophrenia*. New York, NY: Guilford Press.

(2005). *Cognitive Therapy of Schizophrenia*. New York, NY: Guilford Press.

Kirkpatrick, B., Buchanan, R. W., McKenny, P. D., Alphs, L. D., & Carpenter, W. T. (1989). The schedule for the deficit syndrome: an instrument for research in schizophrenia. *Psychiatry Research*, 30(2), 119–123.

Kirkpatrick, B., Strauss, G. P., Nguyen, L. et al. (2010). The brief negative symptom scale: psychometric properties. *Schizophrenia Bulletin*, 37(2), 300–305. doi: 10.1093/schbul/sbq059

Kline, E., & Keshavan, M. (2017). Innovations in first episode psychosis interventions: the case for a "RAISE-Plus" approach. *Schizophrenia Research*, 182(supplement C), 2–3. doi: 10.1016/j.schres.2017.03.035

Klintsova, A. Y., & Greenough, W. T. (1999). Synaptic plasticity in cortical systems. *Current Opinion in Neurobiology*, 9(2), 203–208.

Knöchel, C., Voss, M., Grüter, F. et al. (2015). Omega 3 fatty acids: novel neurotherapeutic targets for cognitive dysfunction in mood disorders and schizophrenia? *Current Neuropharmacology*, 13(5), 663–680.

Kobayashi, M., & Pascual-Leone, A. (2003). Transcranial magnetic stimulation in neurology. *Lancet Neurology*, 2(3), 145–156.

Kohler, C. G., Turner, T. H., Bilker, W. B. et al. (2003). Facial emotion recognition in schizophrenia: intensity effects and error pattern. *American Journal of Psychiatry*, 160(10), 1768–1774. doi: 10.1176/appi.ajp.160.10.1768

Koreen, A. R., Siris, S. G., Chakos, M., & Alvir, J. (1993). Depression in first-episode schizophrenia. *American Journal of Psychiatry, 150*(11), 1643.

Koren, D., Seidman, L. J., Goldsmith, M., & Harvey, P. D. (2006). Real-world cognitive – and metacognitive – dysfunction in schizophrenia: a new approach for measuring (and remediating) more "right stuff". *Schizophrenia Bulletin, 32*(2), 310–326.

Kornell, N., & Bjork, R. A. (2008). Learning concepts and categories: is spacing the "enemy of induction? *Psychological Science, 19*, 585–592.

Krabbendam, L., & Aleman, A. (2003). Cognitive rehabilitation in schizophrenia: a quantitative analysis of controlled studies. *Psychopharmacology (Berl), 169*(3–4), 376–382.

Kraepelin, E., Barclay, R. M., & Robertson, G. M. (1919). *Dementia Praecox and Paraphrenia.* Chicago: Chicago Medical Book Co.

Kurtz, M. M., & Richardson, C. L. (2011). Social cognitive training for schizophrenia: a meta-analytic investigation of controlled research. *Schizophrenia Bulletin, 38*(5), 1092–1104. doi: 10.1093/schbul/sbr036

Lebedev, M. A., & Nicolelis, M. A. (2017). Brain-machine interfaces: from basic science to neuroprostheses and neurorehabilitation. *Physiological Reviews, 97*(2), 767–837.

Lee, H., Dvorak, D., Kao, H. Y. et al. (2012). Early cognitive experience prevents adult deficits in a neurodevelopmental schizophrenia model. *Neuron, 75*(4), 714–724.

Lehrer, D. S., & Lorenz, J. (2014). Anosognosia in schizophrenia: hidden in plain sight. *Innovations in Clinical Neuroscience, 11*(5–6), 10–17.

Leifker, F. R., Patterson, T. L., Heaton, R. K., & Harvey, P. D. (2009). Validating measures of real-world outcome: the results of the VALERO expert survey and RAND panel. *Schizophrenia Bulletin, 37*(2), 334–343. doi: 10.1093/schbul/sbp044

Lett, T. A., Voineskos, A. N., Kennedy, J. L., Levine, B., & Daskalakis, Z. J. (2014). Treating working memory deficits in schizophrenia: a review of the neurobiology. *Biological Psychiatry, 75*(5), 361–370. doi: 10.1016/j.biopsych.2013.07.026

Lewandowski, K. E., Eack, S. M., Hogarty, S. S., Greenwald, D. P., & Keshavan, M. S. (2011). Is cognitive enhancement therapy equally effective for patients with schizophrenia and schizoaffective disorder? *Schizophrenia Research, 125*(2–3), 291–294. doi: 10.1016/j.schres.2010.11.017

Lewandowski, K. E., Ongur, D., & Keshavan, M. S. (2017). Development of novel behavioral interventions in an experimental therapeutics world: challenges, and directions for the future. *Schizophrenia Research.* doi: 10.1016/j.schres.2017.06.010

Lewis, D. A. (2014). Inhibitory neurons in human cortical circuits: substrate for cognitive dysfunction in schizophrenia. *Current Opinion in Neurobiology, 26*(supplement C), 22–26. doi: 10.1016/j.conb.2013.11.003

Liberman, R. P., Massel, H. K., Mosk, M. D., & Wong, S. E. (1985). Social skills training for chronic mental patients. *Psychiatric Services, 36*(4), 396–403. doi: 10.1176/ps.36.4.396

Liddle, P. F. (1987). The symptoms of chronic schizophrenia. A re-examination of the positive-negative dichotomy. *British Journal of Psychiatry, 151*(2), 145–151.

Lieberman, J. A., Papadakis, K., Csernansky, J. et al. (2009). MEM-MD-29 study group. A randomized, placebo-controlled study of memantine as adjunctive treatment in patients with schizophrenia. *Neuropsychopharmacology, 34*(5), 1322–1329.

Linden, M., Hawley, C., Blackwood, B. et al. (2016). Technological aids for the rehabilitation of memory and executive functioning in children and adolescents with acquired brain injury. *Cochrane Database of Systematic Reviews, 7*, CD011020.

Lindenmayer, J. P., & Khan, A. (2011). Galantamine augmentation of long-acting injectable risperidone for cognitive impairments in chronic schizophrenia. *Schizophrenia Research, 125*(2), 267–277. doi: 10.1016/j.schres.2010.08.021

Lindenmayer, J. P., Khan, A., Lachman, H. et al. (2015). COMT genotype and response to cognitive remediation in schizophrenia. *Schizophrenia Research, 168*(1–2), 279–284.

Lindenmayer, J. P., McGurk, S. R., Mueser, K. T. et al. (2008). A randomized controlled trial of cognitive remediation among inpatients with persistent mental illness. *Psychiatric Services*, 59(3), 241–247. doi: 10.1176/appi .ps.59.3.241

Lindenmayer, J. P., Ozog, V. A., Khan, A. et al. (2017). Predictors of response to cognitive remediation in service recipients with severe mental illness. *Psychiatric Rehabilitation Journal*, 40(1), 61–69.

Liu C. H., Keshavan M. S., Tronick E., Seidman L. J. (2015a). Perinatal risks and childhood premorbid indicators of later psychosis: next steps for early psychosocial interventions. *Schizophrenia Bulletin* 41(4):801–16.

Liu, B., Teng, F., Fu, H., et al. (2015b). Excessive intraoperative blood loss independently predicts recurrence of hepatocellular carcinoma after liver transplantation. *BMC Gastroenterology*, 15, 138. doi: 10.1186/ s12876-015-0364-5

Lomo, T. (2003). The discovery of long-term potentiation. *Philosophical Transactions of the Royal Society of London B: Biological Sciences*, 358(1432), 617–620. doi: 10.1098/ rstb.2002.1226

Lysaker, P. H., Dimaggio, G., Buck, K. D., Carcione, A., & Nicolò, G. (2007). Metacognition within narratives of schizophrenia: associations with multiple domains of neurocognition. *Schizophrenia Research*, 93(1), 278–287.

Lysaker, P. H., Dimaggio, G., Carcione, A. et al. (2010). Metacognition and schizophrenia: the capacity for self-reflectivity as a predictor for prospective assessments of work performance over six months. *Schizophrenia Research*, 122(1), 124–130.

Lysaker, P. H., Leonhardt, B. L., Pijnenborg, M. et al. (2014). Metacognition in schizophrenia spectrum disorders: methods of assessment and associations with neurocognition, symptoms, cognitive style and function. *Israel Journal of Psychiatry and Related Sciences*, 51(1), 54–61.

Lysaker, P. H., Vohs, J., Minor, K. S. et al. (2015). Metacognitive deficits in schizophrenia. *Journal of Nervous and Mental Disease*, 203(7), 530–536. doi: 10.1097/nmd.0000000000000323

Maguire, E. A., Gadian, D. G., Johnsrude, I. S. et al. (2000). Navigation-related structural change in the hippocampi of taxi drivers. *Proceedings of the National Academy of Sciences of the United States of America*, 97(8), 4398–4403. doi: 10.1073/pnas.070039597

Manganas, L. N., Zhang, X., Li, Y. et al. (2007). Magnetic resonance spectroscopy identifies neural progenitor cells in the live human brain. *Science*, 318(5852), 980–985. doi: 10.1126/science.1147851

Marjoram, D., Tansley, H., Miller, P. et al. (2005). A theory of mind investigation into the appreciation of visual jokes in schizophrenia. *BMC Psychiatry*, 5(1), 12.

Markham, J. A., & Greenough, W. T. (2004). Experience-driven brain plasticity: beyond the synapse. *Neuron Glia Biology*, 1(4), 351–363. doi: 10.1017/s1740925x05000219

Marshall, M., & Rathbone, J. (2011). Early intervention for psychosis. *Schizophrenia Bulletin*, 37(6), 1111–1114. doi: 10.1093/ schbul/sbr110

Maslow, A. H. (1943). A theory of human motivation. *Psychological Review*, 50(4), 370–396. doi: 10.1037/h0054346

Mathew, I., Gardin, T. M., Tandon, N. et al. (2014). Medial temporal lobe structures and hippocampal subfields in psychotic disorders: findings from the Bipolar-Schizophrenia Network on Intermediate Phenotypes (B-SNIP) study. *JAMA Psychiatry*, 71(7), 769–777.

Mausbach, B. T., Harvey, P. D., Goldman, S. R., Jeste, D. V., & Patterson, T. L. (2007). Development of a brief scale of everyday functioning in persons with serious mental illness. *Schizophrenia Bulletin*, 33(6), 1364–1372.

Mayer, J. D., Salovey, P., Caruso, D. R., & Sitarenios, G. (2003). Measuring emotional intelligence with the MSCEIT V2.0. *Emotion*, 3(1), 97–105. doi: 10.1037/1528-3542.3.1.97

Mayes, A., Montaldi, D., & Migo, E. (2007). Associative memory and the medial temporal lobes. *Trends in Cognitive Sciences*, 11(3), 126–135. doi: 10.1016/j.tics.2006 .12.003

Mayfield, K. H., & Chase, P. N. (2002). The effects of cumulative practice on mathematics problem solving. *Journal of Applied Behavior Analysis*, 35, 105–123.

McDonald, S., Flanagan, S., Rollins, J., & Kinch, J. (2003). TASIT: A new clinical tool for assessing social perception after traumatic brain injury. *Journal of Head Trauma Rehabilitation*, *18*(3), 219–238.

McGhie, A., & Chapman, J. (1961). Disorders of attention and perception in early schizophrenia. *British Journal of Medical Psychology*, *34*, 103–116.

McGrath, J., Saha, S., Welham, J. et al. (2004). A systematic review of the incidence of schizophrenia: the distribution of rates and the influence of sex, urbanicity, migrant status and methodology. *BMC Medicine*, *2*(13), 1–22.

McGurk, S. R. (2005). Cognitive training and supported employment for persons with severe mental illness: one-year results from a randomized controlled trial. *Schizophrenia Bulletin*, *31*(4), 898–909. doi: 10.1093/schbul/sbi037

McGurk, S. R., Mueser, K. T., Xie, H. et al. (2015). Cognitive enhancement treatment for people with mental illness who do not respond to supported employment: a randomized controlled trial. *American Journal of Psychiatry*, *172*(9), 852–861. doi: 10.1176/appi.ajp.2015.14030374

McGurk, S. R., Mueser, K. T., Feldman, K., Wolfe, R., & Pascaris, A. (2007a). Cognitive training for supported employment: 2–3 year outcomes of a randomized controlled trial. *American Journal of Psychiatry*, *164*(3), 437–441.

McGurk, S. R., Twamley, E. W., Sitzer, D. I., McHugo, G. J., & Mueser, K. T. (2007b). A meta-analysis of cognitive remediation in schizophrenia. *American Journal of Psychiatry*, *164*(12), 1791–1802. doi: 10.1176/appi.ajp.2007.07060906

McHugh, R. K., & Barlow, D. H. (2010). The dissemination and implementation of evidence-based psychological treatments: a review of current efforts. *American Psychologist*, *65*(2), 73–84.

McNab, F., Varrone, A., Farde, L., et al. (2009). Changes in cortical dopamine D1 receptor binding associated with cognitive training. *Science*. *323*(5915), 800–2.

Meaney, M. J. (2001). Maternal care, gene expression, and the transmission of individual differences in stress reactivity across generations. *Annual Review of Neuroscience*, *24*(1), 1161–1192.

Mears, R. P., & Spencer, K. M. (2012). Electrophysiological assessment of auditory stimulus-specific plasticity in schizophrenia. *Biological Psychiatry*, *71*(6), 503–511. doi: 10.1016/j.biopsych.2011.12.016

Medalia, A., Erlich, M. D., Soumet-Leman, C., & Saperstein, A. M. (2017). Translating cognitive behavioral interventions from bench to bedside: the feasibility and acceptability of cognitive remediation in research as compared to clinical settings. *Schizophrenia Research*. doi: 10.1016/j.schres.2017.07.044. [Epub ahead of print]

Medalia, A., & Freilich, B. (2008). The Neuropsychological Educational Approach to Cognitive Remediation (NEAR) model: practice principles and outcome studies. *American Journal of Psychiatric Rehabilitation*, *11*(2), 123–143. doi: 10.1080/15487760801963660

Medalia, A., Herlands, T., & Baginsky, C. (2003). Rehab rounds: cognitive remediation in the supportive housing setting. *Psychiatric Services*, *54*(9), 1219–1220. doi: 10.1176/appi.ps.54.9.1219

Medalia, A., Revheim, N., & Casey, M. (2002). Remediation of problem-solving skills in schizophrenia: evidence of a persistent effect. *Schizophrenia Research*, *57*(2–3), 165–171. doi: 10.1016/s0920-9964(01)00293-6

Medalia, A., Revheim, N., & Herlands, T. (2009). *Cognitive Remediation for Psychological Disorders*. New York, NY: Oxford University Press.

Medalia, A., & Saperstein, A. (2011). The role of motivation for treatment success. *Schizophrenia Bulletin*, *37*(supplement 2), S122–S128. doi: 10.1093/schbul/sbr063

Medalia, A., & Saperstein, A. M. (2013). Does cognitive remediation for schizophrenia improve functional outcomes? *Current Opinion in Psychiatry*, *26*, 151–157.

Mervis, J. E., Capizzi, R. J., Boroda, E., & MacDonald III, A. W. (2017). Transcranial direct current stimulation over the dorsolateral prefrontal cortex in schizophrenia: a quantitative review of cognitive outcomes. *Frontiers in Human Neuroscience*, 1–8.

Merzenich, M. M., Jenkins, W. M., Johnston, P. et al. (1996). Temporal processing deficits of language-learning impaired children ameliorated by training. *Science, 271*(5245), 77–81. doi: 10.1126/science.271.5245.77

Mesholam-Gately, R. I., Giuliano, A. J., Goff, K. P., Faraone, S. V., & Seidman, L. J. (2009). Neurocognition in first-episode schizophrenia: a meta-analytic review. *Neuropsychology, 23*(3), 315.

Metz, A., & Albers, B. (2014). What does it take? How federal initiatives can support the implementation of evidence-based programs to improve outcomes for adolescents. *Journal of Adolescent Health, 54*(3), S92–S96.

Michalopoulou, P. G., Lewis, S. W., Drake, R. J. et al. (2015). Modafinil combined with cognitive training: pharmacological augmentation of cognitive training in schizophrenia. *European Neuropsychopharmacology, 25*(8), 1178–1189.

Moore, H., Geyer, M. A., Carter, C. S., & Barch, D. M. (2013). Harnessing cognitive neuroscience to develop new treatments for improving cognition in schizophrenia: CNTRICS selected cognitive paradigms for animal models. *Neuroscience & Biobehavioral Reviews, 37*(9, Part B), 2087–2091. doi: 10.1016/j.neubiorev.2013.09.011

Moritz, S., & Woodward, T. S.. (2007). Metacognitive training in schizophrenia: from basic research to knowledge translation and intervention. *Current Opinion in Psychiatry, 20*(6), 619–625.

Moritz, S., Andreou, C., Schneider, B. C. et al. (2014). Sowing the seeds of doubt: a narrative review on metacognitive training in schizophrenia. *Clinical Psychology Review, 34*(4), 358–366.

Moritz, S., & Woodward, T. S. (2005). Jumping to conclusions in delusional and non-delusional schizophrenic patients. *British Journal of Clinical Psychology, 44*(2), 193–207. doi: 10.1348/014466505x35678

Morrens, M., Hulstijn, W., & Sabbe, B. (2006). Psychomotor slowing in schizophrenia. *Schizophrenia Bulletin, 33*(4), 1038–1053.

Mueller, D. R., Schmidt, S. J., & Roder, V. (2015). One-year randomized controlled trial and follow-up of integrated neurocognitive therapy for schizophrenia outpatients. *Schizophrenia Bulletin, 41*(3), 604–616.

Mueser, K. T., Deavers, F., Penn, D. L., & Cassisi, J. E. (2013). Psychosocial treatments for schizophrenia. *Annual Review of Clinical Psychology, 9*, 465–497.

Mueser, K. T., Penn, D. L., Blanchard, J. J., & Bellack, A. S. (1997). Affect recognition in schizophrenia: a synthesis of findings across three studies. *Psychiatry, 60*(4), 301–308.

Nagarajan, S., Mahncke, H., Salz, T. et al. (1999). Cortical auditory signal processing in poor readers. *Proceedings of the National Academy of Sciences, 96*(11), 6483–6488. doi: 10.1073/pnas.96.11.6483

Nahum, M., Fisher, M., Loewy, R. et al. (2014). A novel, online social cognitive training program for young adults with schizophrenia: a pilot study. *Schizophrenia Research: Cognition, 1*(1), e11–e19. doi: 10.1016/j.scog.2014.01.003

National Institute of Mental Health. (2012). *Recovery After an Initial Schizophrenia Episode: A Research Project of the NIMH* from nimh.nih.gov/health/topics/schizophrenia/raise/index.shtml

Nelson, C. A. (2000). *Neurons to Neighborhoods*. Washington, DC: National Academies Press.

Nestler, E. J., & Hyman, S. E. (2010). Animal models of neuropsychiatric disorders. *Nature Neuroscience, 13*(10), 1161–1169.

Newman, L. S. (2001). What is Social Cognition? Four Basic Approaches and Their Implications for Schizophrenia Research. In P. W. Corrigan & D. L. Penn (Eds.), *Social Cognition and Schizophrenia* (pp. 41–72). Washington, DC: American Psychological Association.

Nitsche, M. A., & Paulus, W. (2000). Excitability changes induced in the human motor cortex by weak transcranial direct current stimulation. *Journal of Physiology, 527 (Pt 3)*, 633–639.

Nuechterlein, K. H., Green, M. F., Kern, R. S. et al. (2008) The MATRICS Consensus Cognitive Battery, part 1: test selection, reliability, and validity. *American Journal of Psychiatry, 165*(2), 203–13.

Nuechterlein, K. H., Ventura J., Subotnik K. L. et al. (2014). Developing a cognitive training strategy for first-episode schizophrenia: integrating bottom-up and top-down approaches. *American Journal of Psychiatric Rehabilitation, 17*, 225–253.

Oberman, L., & Pascual-Leone, A. (2013). Changes in plasticity across the lifespan: cause of disease and target for intervention. *Progress in Brain Research, 207,* 91–120. doi: 10.1016/B978-0-444-63327-9.00016-3

Osborne, A. L., Solowij, N., & Weston-Green, K. (2017). A systematic review of the effect of cannabidiol on cognitive function: relevance to schizophrenia. *Neuroscience & Biobehavioral Reviews, 72*(supplement C), 310–324. doi: 10.1016/j.neubiorev.2016.11.012

Oxley, T., Fitzgerald, P. B., Brown, T. L. et al. (2004). Repetitive transcranial magnetic stimulation reveals abnormal plastic response to premotor cortex stimulation in schizophrenia. *Biological Psychiatry, 56*(9), 628–633. doi: 10.1016/j.biopsych.2004.08.023

Overall, J. E., & Gorham, D. R. (1962). The brief psychiatric rating scale. *Psychological Reports, 10*(3), 799–812.

Papa, M., De Luca, C., Petta, F., Alberghina, L., & Cirillo, G. (2014). Astrocyte-neuron interplay in maladaptive plasticity. *Neuroscience & Biobehavioral Reviews, 42,* 35–54. doi: 10.1016/j.neubiorev.2014.01.010

Papiol, S., Popovic, D., Keeser, D. et al. (2017). Polygenic risk has an impact on the structural plasticity of hippocampal subfields during aerobic exercise combined with cognitive remediation in multi-episode schizophrenia. *Translational Psychiatry, 7*(6), 1–9.

Patterson, T. L., Goldman, S., McKibbin, C. L., Hughs, T., & Jeste, D. V. (2001). UCSD Performance-based skills assessment: development of a new measure of everyday functioning for severely mentally ill adults. *Schizophrenia Bulletin, 27*(2), 235–245.

Patterson, T. L., McKibbin, C., Taylor, M. et al. (2003). Functional Adaptation Skills Training (FAST): a pilot psychosocial intervention study in middle-aged and older patients with chronic psychotic disorders. *American Journal of Geriatric Psychiatry, 11*(1), 17–23. doi: 10.1097/00019442-200301000-00004

Pearlson, G. D., Petty, R. G., Ross, C. A., & Tien, A. Y. (1996). Schizophrenia: a disease of heteromodal association cortex? *Neuropsychopharmacology, 14*(1), 1–17.

Penades, R., Pujol, N., Catalan, R. et al. (2013). Brain effects of cognitive remediation therapy in schizophrenia: a structural and functional neuroimaging study. *Biological Psychiatry, 73*(10), 1015–1023. doi: 10.1016/j.biopsych.2013.01.017

Penn, D., Roberts, D. L., Munt, E. D. et al. (2005). A pilot study of social cognition and interaction training (SCIT) for schizophrenia. *Schizophrenia Research, 80*(2–3), 357–359. doi: 10.1016/j.schres.2005.07.011

Penn, D. L., Corrigan, P. W., Bentall, R. P., Racenstein, J. M., & Newman, L. (1997). Social cognition in schizophrenia. *Psychological Bulletin, 121*(1), 114–132. doi: 10.1037//0033-2909.121.1.114

Perkins, D. O. (2002). Predictors of noncompliance in patients with schizophrenia. *Journal of Clinical Psychiatry, 63*(12), 1121–1128.

Perkins, D. O., Gu, H., Boteva, K., & Lieberman, J. A. (2005). Relationship between duration of untreated psychosis and outcome in first-episode schizophrenia: a critical review and meta-analysis. *American Journal of Psychiatry, 162*(10), 1785–1804. doi: 10.1176/appi.ajp.162.10.1785

Perlman, S. B., & Pelphrey, K. A. (2011). Developing connections for affective regulation: age-related changes in emotional brain connectivity. *Journal of Experimental Child Psychology, 108*(3), 607–620.

Peterson, C., Semmel, A., Von Baeyer, C., et al. (1982). The attributional style questionnaire. *Cognitive Therapy and Research, 6*(3), 287–300.

Peterson, D. E., Beck, S. L., & Keefe, D. M. (2004). Novel therapies. *Seminars in Oncology Nursing, 20*(1), 53–58.

Phillips, M. L., Drevets, W. C., Rauch, S. L., & Lane, R. (2003). Neurobiology of emotion perception I: the neural basis of normal emotion perception. *Biological Psychiatry, 54*(5), 504–514.

Pietrzak, R. H., Olver, J., Norman, T. et al. (2009). A comparison of the CogState schizophrenia battery and the Measurement and Treatment Research to Improve Cognition in Schizophrenia (MATRICS) battery in assessing cognitive impairment in chronic schizophrenia. *Journal of Clinical and Experimental Neuropsychology, 31*(7), 848–859. doi: 10.1080/13803390802592458

Pirttimaki, T. M., & Parri, H. R. (2013). Astrocyte plasticity: implications for synaptic and neuronal activity. *Neuroscientist*, *19*(6), 604–615. doi: 10.1177/1073858413504999

Pittenger, C. (2013). Disorders of memory and plasticity in psychiatric disease. *Dialogues in Clinical Neuroscience*, *15*(4), 455–463.

Popov, T., Jordanov, T., Rockstroh, B. et al. (2011). Specific cognitive training normalizes auditory sensory gating in schizophrenia: a randomized trial. *Biological Psychiatry*, *69*(5), 465–471. doi: 10.1016/j .biopsych.2010.09.028

Powell, S. B., Weber, M., & Geyer, M. A. (2012). Genetic Models of Sensorimotor Gating: Relevance to Neuropsychiatric Disorders. *Current Topics in Behavioral Neuroscience*, *12*, 251–318.

Pratt, J., Winchester, C., Dawson, N., & Morris, B. (2012). Advancing schizophrenia drug discovery: optimizing rodent models to bridge the translational gap. *Nature Reviews Drug Discovery*, *11*, 560–579.

Rabany, L., Deutsch, L., & Levkovitz, Y. (2014). Double-blind, randomized sham controlled study of deep-TMS add-on treatment for negative symptoms and cognitive deficits in schizophrenia. *Journal of Psychopharmacology*, *28*(7), 686–690. doi: 10.1177/0269881114533600

Raffard, S., Gely-Nargeot, M. C., Capdevielle, D., Bayard, S., & Boulenger, J. P. (2009) [Learning potential and cognitive remediation in schizophrenia]. *Encephale*, *35*(4), 353–60.

Ramon y Cajal, S. (1894). The Croonian lecture: la fine structure des centres nerveux. *Proceedings of the Royal Society of London*, *55*, 331–335.

Ramsay, I. S., & MacDonald, A. W. (2015). Brain correlates of cognitive remediation in schizophrenia: activation likelihood analysis shows preliminary evidence of neural target engagement. *Schizophrenia Bulletin*, *41*(6), 1276–1284. doi: 10.1093/ schbul/sbv025

Randolph, C., Tierney, M. C., Mohr, E., & Chase, T. N. (1998). The Repeatable Battery for the Assessment of Neuropsychological Status (RBANS): preliminary clinical validity. *Journal of Clinical and Experimental Neuropsychology*, *20*(3), 310–319.

Rector, N. A., & Beck, A. T. (2012). Cognitive behavioral therapy for schizophrenia: an empirical review Neil A. Rector, PhD and Aaron T. Beck, MD (2001). Reprinted from the Journal of Nervous and Mental Disease. 189, 278–287. *Journal of Nervous and Mental Disease*, *200*(10), 832–839.

Reeder, C., Huddy, V., Cella, M. et al. (2017). A new generation computerised metacognitive cognitive remediation programme for schizophrenia (CIRCuiTS): a randomised controlled trial. *Psychological Medicine*, *47*(15), 2720–2730.

Revell, E. R., Neill, J. C., Harte, M., Khan, Z., & Drake, R. J. (2015). A systematic review and meta-analysis of cognitive remediation in early schizophrenia. *Schizophrenia Research*, *168*(1–2), 213–222. doi: 10.1016/j.schres .2015.08.017

Roberts, D. L., & Penn, D. L. (2009). Social Cognition and Interaction Training (SCIT) for outpatients with schizophrenia: a preliminary study. *Psychiatry Research*, *166*(2–3), 141–147. doi: 10.1016/j.psychres .2008.02.007

Robinson, D. G., Gallego, J. A., John, M. et al. (2015). A randomized comparison of aripiprazole and risperidone for the acute treatment of first-episode schizophrenia and related disorders: 3-month outcomes. *Schizophrenia Bulletin*, *41*(6), 1227–1236.

Robinson, D. G., Woerner, M. G., McMeniman, M., Mendelowitz, A., & Bilder, R. M. (2004). Symptomatic and functional recovery from a first episode of schizophrenia or schizoaffective disorder. *American Journal of Psychiatry*, *161*(3), 473–479. doi: 10.1176/ appi.ajp.161.3.473

Roder, V. (2006). Integrated Psychological Therapy (IPT) for schizophrenia: is it effective? *Schizophrenia Bulletin*, *32*(supplement 1), S81–S93. doi: 10.1093/ schbul/sbl021

Rogasch, N. C., & Fitzgerald, P. B. (2013). Assessing cortical network properties using TMS–EEG. *Human Brain Mapping*, *34*(7), 1652–1669.

Rosanova, M., & Ulrich, D. (2005). Pattern-specific associative long-term potentiation induced by a sleep spindle-related spike train. *Journal of Neuroscience*, *25*(41), 9398–9405. doi: 10.1523/ JNEUROSCI.2149-05.2005

Rosenthal, M., & Braant, S. (2003). Benefits of adjunct modafinil in an open-label, pilot study in patients with schizophrenia. *Schizophrenia Research, 60*(1), 301.

Rossi S., Cappa, S. F., Babiloni, C. et al. (2001). Prefrontal [correction of Prefontal] cortex in long-term memory: an "interference" approach using magnetic stimulation. *Nature Neuroscience, 4*(9), 48–52.

Rund, B. R. (1998). A review of longitudinal studies of cognitive function in schizophrenia patients. *Schizophrenia Bulletin, 24*(3), 425–435.

Ruse S. A., Harvey, P. D., Davis, V. G. et al. (2014). Virtual reality functional capacity assessment in schizophrenia: Preliminary data regarding feasibility and correlations with cognitive and functional capacity performance. Schizophrenia Research: *Cognition, 1*(1), pp. e21–e26.

Russell, T. A., Chu, E., & Phillips, M. L. (2006). A pilot study to investigate the effectiveness of emotion recognition remediation in schizophrenia using the micro-expression training tool. *British Journal of Clinical Psychology, 45*(4), 579–583. doi: 10.1348/014466505x90866

Ryan, R. M., & Deci, E. L. (2000). Intrinsic and extrinsic motivations: classic definitions and new directions. *Contemporary Educational Psychology, 25*(1), 54–67.

Sabbag, S., Twamley, E. M., Vella, L. et al. (2011). Assessing everyday functioning in schizophrenia: not all informants seem equally informative. *Schizophrenia Research, 131*(1–3), 250–255. doi: 10.1016/j.schres.2011.05.003

Sacks, S., Fisher, M., Garrett, C. et al. (2013). Combining computerized social cognitive training with neuroplasticity-based auditory training in schizophrenia. *Clinical Schizophrenia & Related Psychoses, 7*(2), 78–86A. doi: 10.3371/csrp.safi.012513

Saha, S., Chant, D., Welham, J., & McGrath, J. (2005). A systematic review of the prevalence of schizophrenia. *PLoS Medicine, 2*(5), e141.

Sahakian, B. J., Morris, R. G., Evenden, J. L. et al. (1988). A comparative study of visuospatial memory and learning in Alzheimer-type dementia and Parkinson's disease. *Brain, 111*(3), 695–718.

Salovey, P., & Mayer, J. D. (1990). Emotional intelligence. *Imagination, Cognition and Personality, 9*(3), 185–211. doi: 10.2190/dugg-p24e-52wk-6cdg

Samara, M. T., Leucht, C., Leeflang, M. M. et al. (2015). Early improvement as a predictor of later response to antipsychotics in schizophrenia: a diagnostic test review. *American Journal of Psychiatry, 172*(7), 617–629.

Sandoval, L. R., González, B. L., Stone, W. S. et al. (2017). Effects of peer social interaction on performance during computerized cognitive remediation therapy in patients with early course schizophrenia: a pilot study. *Schizophrenia Research.* doi: 10.1016/j.schres.2017.08.049. [Epub ahead of print]

Saperstein, A. M., & Medalia, A. (2015). The role of motivation in cognitive remediation for people with schizophrenia. *Current Topics in Behavioral Neurosciences, 172*, 533–546.

Sartory, G., Zorn, C., Groetzinger, G., & Windgassen, K. (2005). Computerized cognitive remediation improves verbal learning and processing speed in schizophrenia. *Schizophrenia Research, 75*(2–3), 219–223. doi: 10.1016/j.schres.2004.10.004

Satogami, K., Takahashi, S., Yamada, S., Ukai, S., & Shinosaki, K. (2017). Omega-3 fatty acids related to cognitive impairment in patients with schizophrenia. *Schizophrenia Research: Cognition, 9*, 8–12.

Savla, G. N., Vella, L., Armstrong, C. C., Penn, D. L., & Twamley, E. W. (2012). Deficits in domains of social cognition in schizophrenia: a meta-analysis of the empirical evidence. *Schizophrenia Bulletin, 39*(5), 979–992. doi: 10.1093/schbul/sbs080

Saxe, R., & Kanwisher, N. (2003). People thinking about thinking people. The role of the temporo-parietal junction in "theory of mind". *Neuroimage, 19*(4), 1835–1842.

Schmidt, S. J., Mueller, D. R., & Roder, V. (2011). Social cognition as a mediator variable between neurocognition and functional outcome in schizophrenia: empirical review and new results by structural equation modeling. *Schizophrenia Bulletin, 37*(supplement 2), S41–S54.

Schneider, L. C., & Struening, E. L. (1983). SLOF: a behavioral rating scale for assessing the mentally ill. *Social Work Research and Abstracts, 19*(3), 9–21. doi: 10.1093/swra/19.3.9

Schoenwald, S. K., Kelleher, K., & Weisz, J. R. (2008). The research network on youth mental health. Building bridges to evidence-based practice: The MacArthur Foundation Child System and Treatment Enhancement Projects (Child STEPs). *Administration and Policy in Mental Health and Mental Health Services Research, 35*(1–2), 66–72.

Scoriels, L., Barnett, J. H., Soma, P. K., Sahakian, B. J., & Jones, P. B. (2012). Effects of modafinil on cognitive functions in first episode psychosis. *Psychopharmacology (Berl.), 220*, 249–258.

Seidman, L. J., Giuliano, A. J., Meyer, E. C. et al. (2010). Neuropsychology of the prodrome to psychosis in the NAPLS consortium: relationship to family history and conversion to psychosis. *Archives of General Psychiatry, 67*(6), 578–588.

Sergi, M. J., Fiske, A. P., Horan, W. P. et al. (2009). Development of a measure of relationship perception in schizophrenia. *Psychiatry Research, 166*(1), 54–62. doi: 10.1016/j.psychres.2008.03.010

Sergi, M. J., Rassovsky, Y., Nuechterlein, K. H., & Green, M. F. (2006). Social perception as a mediator of the influence of early visual processing on functional status in schizophrenia. *American Journal of Psychiatry, 163*(3), 448–454.

Sergi, M. J., Rassovsky, Y., Widmark, C. et al. (2007). Social cognition in schizophrenia: relationships with neurocognition and negative symptoms. *Schizophrenia Research, 90*(1–3), 316–324.

Shah, J. L., Tandon, N., Montrose, D. M. et al. (2017). Clinical psychopathology in youth at familial high risk for psychosis. *Early Intervention in Psychiatry.* doi: 10.1111/eip.12480. [Epub ahead of print]

Shashi, V., Harrell, W., Eack, S. et al. (2015). Social cognitive training in adolescents with chromosome 22q11.2 deletion syndrome: feasibility and preliminary effects of the intervention. *Journal of Intellectual Disability Research, 59*(10), 902–913. doi: 10.1111/jir.12192

Shenton, M. E., Kikinis, R., Jolesz, F. A. et al. (1992). Abnormalities of the left temporal lobe and thought disorder in schizophrenia: a quantitative magnetic resonance imaging study. *New England Journal of Medicine, 327*(9), 604–612.

Silver, H., Goodman, C., Knoll, G., & Isakov, V. (2004). Brief emotion training improves recognition of facial emotions in chronic schizophrenia. A pilot study. *Psychiatry Research, 128*(2), 147–154. doi: 10.1016/j.psychres .2004.06.002

Silverstein, S. M., Hatashita-Wong, M., Solak, B. A. et al. (2005). Effectiveness of a two-phase cognitive rehabilitation intervention for severely impaired schizophrenia patients. *Psychological Medicine, 35*(6), 829–837.

Singh, J., Kour, K., & Jayaram, M. B. (2012). Acetylcholinesterase inhibitors for schizophrenia. *Cochrane Database of Systematic Reviews, 18*(1), CD007967. doi: 10.1002/14651858.CD007967 .pub2

Siskind, D., McCartney, L., Goldschlager, R., & Kisely, S. (2016). Clozapine v. first- and second-generation antipsychotics in treatment-refractory schizophrenia: systematic review and meta-analysis. *British Journal of Psychiatry, 209*(5), 385–392. doi: 10.1192/bjp.bp.115.177261

Skevington, S. M., Lotfy, M., & O'Connell, K. A. (2004). The World Health Organization's WHOQOL-BREF quality of life assessment: psychometric properties and results of the international field trial. A report from the WHOQOL Group. *Quality of Life Research, 13*(2), 299–310. doi: 10.1023/b:q ure.0000018486.91360.00

Sliwinski, M. J., Mogle, J. A., Hyun, J. et al. (2016). Reliability and validity of ambulatory cognitive assessments. *Assessment, 5*(1), 14–30. doi: 1073191116643164

Spaulding, W. D. (1992). Design prerequisites for research on cognitive therapy for schizophrenia. *Schizophrenia Bulletin, 18*(1), 39.

Spencer, K. M., Nestor, P. G., Perlmutter, R. et al. (2004). Neural synchrony indexes disordered perception and cognition in schizophrenia. *Proceedings of the National Academy of Sciences of the United States of America, 101*(49), 17288–17293.

Squire, L. R., & Zola-Morgan, S. (1991). The medial temporal lobe memory system. *Science, 253*(5026), 1380.

Srihari, V. H., Shah, J., & Keshavan, M. S. (2012). Is early intervention for psychosis feasible and effective? *Psychiatric Clinics of North America*, *35*(3), 613–631.

Stahnisch, F. W., & Nitsch, R. (2002). Santiago Ramon y Cajal's concept of neuronal plasticity: the ambiguity lives on. *Trends in Neurosciences*, *25*(11), 589–591.

Stein, L. I. (1980). Alternative to mental hospital treatment. *Archives of General Psychiatry*, *37*(4), 392. doi: 10.1001/archpsyc.1980.01780170034003

Stern, Y. (2012). Cognitive reserve in ageing and Alzheimer's disease. *Lancet Neurology*, *11*(11), 1006–1012. doi: 10.1016/s1474-4422(12)70191-6

Stone, W. S., Seidman, L. J., Wojcik, J. D., & Green, A. I. (2003). Glucose effects on cognition in schizophrenia. *Schizophrenia Research*, *62*(1), 93–103.

Stovell, D., Morrison, A. P., Panayiotou, M., & Hutton, P. (2016). Shared treatment decision-making and empowerment-related outcomes in psychosis: systematic review and meta-analysis. *British Journal of Psychiatry*, *209*(1), 23–28.

Subramaniam, K., Luks, T. L., Fisher, M. et al. (2012). Computerized cognitive training restores neural activity within the reality monitoring network in schizophrenia. *Neuron*, *73*(4), 842–853. doi: 10.1016/j.neuron.2011.12.024

Swerdlow, N. R., & Light, G. A. (2016). Animal models of deficient sensorimotor gating in schizophrenia: are they still relevant? *Current Topics in Behavioral Neurosciences*, *28*, 305–325.

Szymanski, L., & King, B. H. (1999). Practice parameters for the assessment and treatment of children, adolescents, and adults with mental retardation and comorbid mental disorders. *Journal of the American Academy of Child & Adolescent Psychiatry*, *38*(12), 5S–31S. doi: 10.1016/s0890-8567(99)80002-1

Tacchino, A., Pedullà, L., Bonzano, L. et al. (2015). A new app for at-home cognitive training: description and pilot testing on patients with multiple sclerosis. *JMIR mHealth and uHealth*, *3*(3), e85.

Takesian, A. E., & Hensch, T. K. (2013). Balancing plasticity/stability across brain development. *Progress in Brain Research*, *207*, 3–34. doi: 10.1016/B978-0-444-63327-9.00001-1

Tamminen, J., Payne, J. D., Stickgold, R., Wamsley, E. J., & Gaskell, M. G. (2010). Sleep spindle activity is associated with the integration of new memories and existing knowledge. *Journal of Neuroscience*, *30*(43), 14356–14360.

Tamminga, C. A., Stan, A. D., & Wagner, A. D. (2010). The hippocampal formation in schizophrenia. *American Journal of Psychiatry*, *167*(10), 1178–1193.

Tandon, R., Nasrallah, H. A., & Keshavan, M. S. (2010). Schizophrenia, "Just the Facts" 5. Treatment and prevention. Past, present, and future. *Schizophrenia Research*, *122*(1), 1–23.

Tcheremissine, O. V., Rossman, W. E., Castro, M. A., & Gardner, D. R. (2014). Conducting clinical research in community mental health settings: opportunities and challenges. *World Journal of Psychiatry*, *4*(3), 49–55.

Thermenos, H., Keshavan, M., Juelich, R. et al. (2013). A review of neuroimaging studies of young relatives of individuals with schizophrenia: a developmental perspective from schizotaxia to schizophrenia. *American Journal of Medical Genetics Part B: Neuropsychiatric Genetics*, *162*(7), 604–635.

Thiede, K. W., Anderson, M., & Therriault, D. (2003). Accuracy of metacognitive monitoring affects learning of texts. *Journal of Educational Psychology*, *95*(1), 66–73.

Thoma, P., & Daum, I. (2008). Working memory and multi-tasking in paranoid schizophrenia with and without comorbid substance use disorder. *Addiction*, *103*(5), 774–786.

Thompson, P. M., Vidal, C., Giedd, J. N. et al. (2001). Mapping adolescent brain change reveals dynamic wave of accelerated gray matter loss in very-early-onset schizophrenia. *Proceedings of the National Academy of Sciences*, *98*(20), 11650–11655.

Tononi, G., & Cirelli, C. (2014). Sleep and the price of plasticity: from synaptic and cellular homeostasis to memory consolidation and integration. *Neuron*, *81*(1), 12–34. doi: 10.1016/j.neuron.2013.12.025

Torous, J., Onnela, J. P., & Keshavan, M. (2017). New dimensions and new tools to realize the potential of RDoC: digital phenotyping via smartphones and connected devices. *Translational Psychiatry*, *7*(3), e1053.

Torous, J., Staples, P., Fenstermacher, E., Dean, J., & Keshavan, M. (2016). Barriers, benefits, and beliefs of brain training smartphone apps: an Internet survey of younger US consumers. *Frontiers in Human Neuroscience, 20*(10), 180. doi: 10.3389/fnhum.2016.00180

Tse, S., Davidson, L., Chung, K. F., Ng, K. L., & Yu, C. H. (2014). Differences and similarities between functional and personal recovery in an Asian population: a cluster analytic approach. *Psychiatry: Interpersonal and Biological Processes, 77*(1), 41–56.

Tullis, J. G., & Benjamin, A. S. (2011). On the effectiveness of self-paced learning. *Journal of Memory and Language, 64*(2), 109–118.

Turner, D. C., Clark, L., Pomarol-Clotet, E. et al. (2004). Modafinil improves cognition and attentional set shifting in patients with chronic schizophrenia. *Neuropsychopharmacology, 29*(7), 1363–1373.

Twamley, E. W., Burton, C. Z., & Vella, L. (2011). Compensatory cognitive training for psychosis: who benefits? Who stays in treatment? *Schizophrenia Bulletin, 37*(supplement 2), S55–62.

Twamley, E. W., Vella, L., Burton, C. Z., Heaton, R. K., & Jeste, D. V. (2012). Compensatory cognitive training for psychosis: effects in a randomized controlled trial. *Journal of Clinical Psychiatry, 73*(9), 1212–1219.

Velligan, D. I., Bow-Thomas, C. C., Huntzinger, C. et al. (2000). Randomized controlled trial of the use of compensatory strategies to enhance adaptive functioning in outpatients with schizophrenia. *American Journal of Psychiatry, 157*(8), 1317–1323.

Velligan, D. I., Roberts, D., Mintz, J. et al. (2015). A randomized pilot study of MOtiVation and Enhancement (MOVE) Training for negative symptoms in schizophrenia. *Schizophrenia Research, 165*(2), 175–180.

Ventura, J., Cienfuegos, A., Boxer, O., & Bilder, R. (2008). Clinical global impression of cognition in schizophrenia (CGI-CogS): reliability and validity of a co-primary measure of cognition. *Schizophrenia Research, 106*(1), 59–69. doi: 10.1016/j.schres.2007.07.025

Ventura, J., Green, M. F., Shaner, A., & Liberman, R. P. (1993). Training and quality assurance with the brief psychiatric rating scale: the drift busters. *International Journal of Methods in Psychiatric Research, 3*(4), 221–244.

Ventura, J., Reise, S. P., Keefe, R. S. et al. (2010). Nuechterlein, K.H., Seidman, L.J. and Bilder, R.M., 2010. The Cognitive Assessment Interview (CAI): development and validation of an empirically derived, brief interview-based measure of cognition. *Schizophrenia Research, 121*(1–3), 24–31.

Ventura, J., Reise, S. P., Keefe, R. S. et al. (2013). The Cognitive Assessment Interview (CAI): reliability and validity of a brief interview-based measure of cognition. *Schizophrenia Bulletin, 39*(3), 583–591.

Vinogradov, S., Fisher, M., Holland, C. et al. (2009). Is serum brain-derived neurotrophic factor a biomarker for cognitive enhancement in schizophrenia? *Biological Psychiatry, 66*(6), 549–553. doi: 10.1016/j.biopsych.2009.02.017

Vita, A., Deste, G., De Peri, L. et al. (2013). Predictors of cognitive and functional improvement and normalization after cognitive remediation in patients with schizophrenia. *Schizophrenia Research, 150*(1), 51–57.

Vizi, E. S. (1979). Presynaptic modulation of neurochemical transmission. *Progress in Neurobiology, 12*(3–4), 181–290.

Volkow, N. D. (2009). Substance use disorders in schizophrenia–clinical implications of comorbidity. *Schizophrenia Bulletin, 35*(3), 469–472. doi: 10.1093/schbul/sbp016

Wallace, C. J., & Liberman, R. P. (1985). Social skills training for patients with schizophrenia: a controlled clinical trial. *Psychiatry Research, 15*(3), 239–247. doi: 10.1016/0165-1781(85)90081-2

Wamsley, E. J., Tucker, M. A., Shinn, A. K. et al. (2012). Reduced sleep spindles and spindle coherence in schizophrenia: mechanisms of impaired memory consolidation? *Biological Psychiatry, 71*(2), 154–161. doi: 10.1016/j.biopsych.2011.08.008

Ward, J. (2007). We are all Larry David: Curb Your Enthusiasm and Psychology. *The Newyorker.* October 29, 2007 Issue

Wechsler, D. (1981). *Wechsler Adult Intelligence Scale-Revised.* San Antonio, TX: Psychological Corp.

Weisz, J. R., Ugueto, A. M., Cheron, D. M., & Herren, J. (2013). Evidence-based youth psychotherapy in the mental health ecosystem. *Journal of Clinical Child & Adolescent Psychology, 42*(2), 274–286.

Whoqol (1998). Development of the World Health Organization WHOQOL-BREF quality of life assessment. *Psychological Medicine, 28*(3), 551–558.

Wiers, R. W., Gladwin, T. E., Hofmann, W., Salemink, E., & Ridderinkhof, K. R. (2013). Cognitive bias modification and cognitive control training in addiction and related psychopathology. *Clinical Psychological Science, 1*(2), 192–212. doi: 10.1177/2167702612466547

Wilk, C. M., Gold, J. M., Bartko, J. J., et al. (2002). Test-retest stability of the Repeatable Battery for the Assessment of Neuropsychological Status in schizophrenia. *American Journal of Psychiatry, 159*(5), 838–44.

Wojtalik, J. A., Eack, S. M., Pollock, B. G., & Keshavan, M. S. (2012). Prefrontal gray matter morphology mediates the association between serum anticholinergicity and cognitive functioning in early course schizophrenia. *Psychiatry Research, 204*(2–3), 61–67.

Wölwer, W., Frommann, N., Halfmann, S. et al. (2005). Remediation of impairments in facial affect recognition in schizophrenia: efficacy and specificity of a new training program. *Schizophrenia Research, 80*(2–3), 295–303. doi: 10.1016/j.schres.2005.07.018

Woodberry, K. A., Giuliano, A. J., & Seidman, L. J. (2008). Premorbid IQ in schizophrenia: a meta-analytic review. *American Journal of Psychiatry, 165*(5), 579–587.

Woodward, N. D., Purdon, S. E., Meltzer, H. Y., & Zald, D. H. (2005). A meta-analysis of neuropsychological change to clozapine, olanzapine, quetiapine, and risperidone in schizophrenia. *International Journal of Neuropsychopharmacology, 8*(3), 457–472.

World Health Organization. (1996). *WHOQOL-BREF: Introduction, Administration, Scoring and Generic Version of the Assessment: Field Trial Version.* Geneva: World Health Organization.

Wu, C., Dagg, P., Molgat, C. (2014). A pilot study to measure cognitive impairment in patients with severe schizophrenia with the Montreal Cognitive Assessment (MoCA). *Schizophrenia Research, 158*(1–3), 151–5.

Wunderink, L., Nieboer, R. M., Wiersma, D., Sytema, S., & Nienhuis, F. J. (2013). Recovery in remitted first-episode psychosis at 7 years of follow-up of an early dose reduction/discontinuation or maintenance treatment strategy: long-term follow-up of a 2-year randomized clinical trial. *JAMA Psychiatry, 70*(9), 913–920.

Wykes, T., Brammer, M., Mellers, J. et al. (2002). Effects on the brain of a psychological treatment: cognitive remediation therapy. *British Journal of Psychiatry, 181*(2), 144–152.

Wykes, T., Huddy, V., Cellard, C., McGurk, S. R., & Czobor, P. (2011). A meta-analysis of cognitive remediation for schizophrenia: methodology and effect sizes. *American Journal of Psychiatry, 168*(5), 472–485. doi: 10.1176/appi.ajp.2010.10060855

Wykes, T., & Reeder, C. (2005). *Cognitive Remediation Therapy for Schizophrenia: An Introduction.* New York, NY: Brunner-Routledge.

Wykes, T., Reeder, C., Corner, J., Williams, C., & Everitt, B. (1999). The effects of neurocognitive remediation on executive processing in patients with schizophrenia. *Schizophrenia Bulletin, 25*(2), 291–307. doi: 10.1093/oxfordjournals.schbul.a033379

Wykes, T., Reeder, C., Williams, C. et al. (2003). Are the effects of cognitive remediation therapy (CRT) durable? Results from an exploratory trial in schizophrenia. *Schizophrenia Research, 61*(2–3), 163–174.

Wykes, T., Reeder, C., Landau, S. et al. (2007). Cognitive remediation therapy in schizophrenia. *British Journal of Psychiatry, 190*(5), 421–427.

Yamaguchi, S., Sato, S., Horio, N. et al. (2017). Cost-effectiveness of cognitive remediation and supported employment for people with mental illness: a randomized controlled trial. *Psychological Medicine, 47*(1), 53–65.

Zhang, J. P., Gallego, J. A., Robinson, D. G. et al. (2013). Efficacy and safety of individual second-generation vs. first-generation antipsychotics in first-episode psychosis: a systematic review and meta-analysis. *International Journal of Neuropsychopharmacology, 16*(6), 1205–1218.

Zortea, K., Franco, V. C., Guimarães, P., & Belmonte-de-Abreu, P. S. (2016). Resveratrol supplementation did not improve cognition in patients with schizophrenia: results from a randomized clinical trial. *Frontiers in Psychiatry, 7*(159).

Zubin, J., & Spring, B. (1977). Vulnerability – a new view of schizophrenia. *Journal of Abnormal Psychology, 86*(2), 103–126.

Index